Kirby I. Bland • Michael G. Sarr
Markus W. Büchler • Attila Csendes
Oliver James Garden • John Wong
(Editors)

Endocrine Surgery

Handbooks in General Surgery

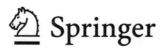 Springer

Editors

Kirby I. Bland
University of Alabama
Birmingham
Department of Surgery
Birmingham, Alabama
USA

Michael G. Sarr
Mayo Clinic
Division of Gastroenterologic &
General Surgery
Rochester, Minnesota
USA

Markus W. Büchler
Universitätsklinikum Heidelberg
Chirurgische Klinik
Abt. Allgemeine, Viszerale und
Unfallchirurgie
Heidelberg
Germany

Attila Csendes
University of Chile
Clinical Hospital
Department of Surgery
Santiago
Chile

Oliver James Garden
University of Edinburgh
Royal Infirmary
Department of Surgery
Edinburgh
United Kingdom

John Wong
Queen Mary Hospital
Department of Surgery
Hong Kong

ISBN 978-1-84996-446-3   e-ISBN 978-1-84996-447-0
DOI 10.1007/978-1-84996-447-0
Springer London Dordrecht Heidelberg New York

British Library Cataloguing in Publication Data
A catalogue record for this book is available from the British Library

Library of Congress Control Number: 2010937966

Cover design: eStudioCalamar Figueres/Berlin

Printed on acid-free paper

Springer is part of Springer Science+Business Media (www.springer.com)

Preface

The editors designed the original textbook, *General Surgery: Principles and International Practice*, from which this shorter paperback monograph on endocrine surgery was taken to be an accessible, concise, and state-of-the-art volume that explores and documents evolutionary principles in the practice of surgery. This work is aimed at the general surgeon and the resident in training. The scientific community continues to witness extraordinary advances in the therapy of both benign and malignant surgical diseases of various organ sites. Much of this progress has been evident over the past decade with new concepts and techniques of management that allow the surgeon to integrate this discipline with medicine, pharmacology, immunology, biostatistics, pathology, genetics, medical and radiation oncology, and diagnostic radiology and imaging. Further, each of these major disciplines contributes a small component for the diagnostic and therapeutic approaches to clinical care; hence the comprehensive planning, integration, and provision of patient care throughout the preoperative, intraoperative, and postoperative phases of care remains essential in the successful practice of our specialty.

The editors acknowledge that the aim of this work is to provide an illustrative, instructive, and comprehensive review that depicts the rationale of basic operative principles essential to surgical therapy. In organizing this monograph, the editors chose authors renowned in the disciplines for illustrating, forming, and depicting in a comprehensive fashion the surgical therapy expectant for metabolic, infectious, endocrine, and neoplastic abnormalities in adult and pediatric patients **from**

a truly international and multi-continental perspective. The editors and authors were chosen carefully from across geographies and also from multi-cultural and diverse locations. While the authors consider this text to be inclusive regarding the technical and operative conditions for perioperative care in this field, its purpose should not be intended to replace standard textbooks of surgery nor should it be considered complete in its coverage of pathophysiologic disorders. In contrast, this monograph is organized to familiarize practicing surgeons, residents, and fellows with state-of-the-art surgical principles and techniques essential to contemporary practice. Therefore, the tenor of this monograph on endocrine surgery has been developed to coexist with other major surgical reference texts that are dedicated—some in more comprehensive fashion—to the therapy of individual organs of systemic diseases. This monograph is much more a "working text" for the practicing surgeon with emphasis on diagnosis and treatment of endocrine disorders. Along with this monograph, nine other paperback monographs are available and focus on the general principles of surgery, trauma, critical care, esophagus and stomach, small bowel, colorectal, liver and biliary, pancreas and spleen, and oncology, all adapted from the primary text-book—*General Surgery: Principles and International Practice*.

The chapters in this monograph on surgery of the esophagus and stomach include a condensed bibliography of highly selective journal articles, reviews, and text. In this manner of attempting to be concise, we hope to provide a precise focus for the education of the reader relative to accepted surgical principles involved in patient care. Moreover, the editors have sought to provide a counterpoint view for the selection of therapy by presenting at the opening of each chapter a list of "Pearls and Pitfalls" that highlight particular concerns or controversies. The chapters provide pertinent, though not exhaustive, summaries of anatomy and physiology, a history of surgical illness, and stages of operative approaches with relevant technical considerations outlined in an easily understandable manner. Complications are reviewed when appropriate for the organ system, diseases, and problem. The text is supported amply by line drawings and photographs that depict anatomic or technical principles. The editors have made every attempt to minimize duplicative or repetitive discussions except when controversial or state-of-the-art issues are presented. Moreover, the editors have attempted to ensure that accurate presentations and illustrations depict properly the most complex problems confronted by the general surgeon.

Finally, in an attempt to address advances in contemporary concepts, the text has been organized to address in detail expeditious, safe, and anatomically accurate operations and incorporate standard as well as evolving surgical principles and techniques. These principles have been tested in the clinics of valid scientific knowledge and are well supported by the time-tested approaches that have been provided by practicing surgeons. The editors are excited to be able to respond to the challenge of developing a truly international text and are indeed hopeful that our readers will find this focused monograph on endocrine surgery to be a repository of insight, useful, and timely information.

Kirby I. Bland
Michael G. Sarr
Markus W. Büchler
Attila Csendes
Oliver James Garden
John Wong

Contents

Contributors

Göran Åkerström, MD, PhD
Professor, Department of Surgical Sciences,
University Hospital, Uppsala, Sweden

Herbert Chen, MD, FACS
Associate Professor, Department of Surgery,
University of Wisconsin, Madison, WI, USA

Orlo H. Clark, MD, FACS
Professor, Department of Surgery,
UCSF/Mt. Zion Medical Center, San Francisco, CA, USA

Henning Dralle, MD, FRCS
Professor of Surgery and Chairman Department of General,
Visceral and Vascular Surgery, Martin Luther University,
Halle-Wittenberg Halle, Germany

Quan-Yang Duh, MD
Professor of Surgery Department of Surgical Service,
University of California-San Francisco,
Veterans Affairs Medical Center, San Francisco,
CA, USA

Volker Fendrich, MD
Assistant Physician, Department of Visceral,
Thoracic, and Vascular Surgery, University of Marburg,
Marburg, Germany

Per Hellman, MD, PhD
Associate Professor, Department of Surgical Sciences,
University Hospital, Uppsala, Sweden

James A. Lee, MD
Assistant Professor, Division of Endocrine Surgery,
Department of Surgery, Mt. Zion Medical Center,
San Francisco, CA, USA

Chung-Yau Lo, MBBC(HK), MS(HK), FRCSC (Edin.), FACS
Chief of Endocrine Surgery, Department of Surgery,
University of Hong Kong Medical Centre,
Queen Mary Hospital, Hong Kong, China

Andreas Machens, MD
Associate Professor of Surgery, Department of General,
Visceral, and Vascular Surgery, Martin Luther University,
Halle-Wittenberg Halle, Germany

Matthias Rothmund, MD, FACS
Chief and Professor, Department of Visceral,
Thoracic, and Vascular Surgery,
University of Marburg, Marburg, Germany

Takashi Uruno, MD
Chief and Professor, Department of Surgery,
UCSF Medical Center at Mt. Zion, San Francisco,
CA, USA

Malcolm H. Wheeler, MD, FRCS
Retired Professor of Endocrine Surgery,
University Hospital of Wales, Cardiff, UK

1
Goiter and Nontoxic Benign Thyroid Conditions

Malcolm H. Wheeler

Pearls and Pitfalls

- Iodine deficiency is a major health problem worldwide affecting approximately 2 billion people, and is causative of endemic goiter in more than 740 million.
- Iodine added to the diet is preventative.
- Diffuse goiter may regress with thyroxine medication.
- Thyroidectomy may be indicated for larger, unresponsive goiters producing compression symptoms or cosmetic effects.
- Palpable thyroid nodules occur in approximately 4% of the US population, the majority of which (90%) are benign and occur in the euthyroid, asymptomatic patient.
- Clinical assessment and investigation are directed toward distinguishing between the benign and malignant nodule.
- Risk factors for malignancy include family history of thyroid cancer, previous neck irradiation, age, physical characteristics of lesion (e.g., size, consistency/fixation), and any associated lymphadenopathy or recurrent laryngeal nerve palsy.
- A solitary nodule in a child under 14 years of age has a 50% chance of being malignant.
- Fine needle aspiration (FNA) biopsy is the single most valuable diagnostic test in the evaluation of thyroid nodules.

K.I. Bland et al. (eds.), *Endocrine Surgery*,
DOI: 10.1007/978-1-84996-447-0_1,
© Springer-Verlag London Limited 2011

- Operative treatment of a thyroid nodule requires at least a complete unilateral thyroid lobectomy including isthmus and pyramidal lobe.
- Operative treatment of multinodular goiter may require unilateral lobectomy with contralateral (partial) resection, although many patients with bilateral disease are best treated by total thyroidectomy and thyroxine replacement.
- Retrosternal goiter generally requires resection; most can be excised through a cervical incision, with only a few (<1%) requiring sternotomy.
- Autoimmune thyroiditis responds typically to thyroxine treatment; risk of lymphoma must be considered when a nodule in a Hashimoto's gland changes in size or consistency.
- Thyroglossal cyst requires total excision including the central portion of the hyoid bone (Sistrunk procedure).

Introduction

The term goiter (L. guttur, throat) is used as a general term to indicate enlargement of the thyroid gland. Classification of goiter may be based on a range of characteristics which include functional, morphologic, anatomic, or pathologic features (Table 1.1).

Simple Goiter

Endemic

The term endemic goiter is used when more than 10% of the population in a defined geographic area have thyroid enlargement. The most common etiology is iodine deficiency, which affects approximately 2 billion people worldwide, resulting in more than 740 million cases of endemic goiter in 13% of the world's population. Predominant locations of endemic goiter

TABLE 1.1. Classification of goiter.

Simple goiter (endemic or sporadic)	Diffuse hyperplastic goiter
	Nodular goiter
Neoplastic goiter	Benign
	Malignant
Toxic goiter	Diffuse (Graves' disease)
	Toxic multinodular goiter
	Toxic solitary nodule
Thyroiditis	Subacute (lymphocytic-de Quervain's)
	Autoimmune (Hashimoto's)
	Riedel's
	Acute suppurative
Miscellaneous	Dyshormonogenesis (e.g. Pendred's)
	Chronic bacterial infection
	(e.g. tuberculosis, syphilis or actinomycosis)
	Amyloidosis
	Ectopic thyroid

include mountainous regions such as the Alps, Andes, and Himalayas, and in lowland regions, particularly Central Africa. Lesser degrees of iodine deficiency persist in several areas of Europe, perhaps most interestingly in Germany, where there is no general policy of salt iodization.

Inadequate iodine intake (adequate daily requirement 100–200 μg) results in decreased synthesis of thyroid hormone, a compensatory increase in TSH secretion, and an increased production of T3 relative to T4. The initial pathologic and clinical effects of increased TSH stimulation are a soft and diffuse enlargement of the thyroid, especially in the young. Fluctuating levels of stimulation result eventually in nodule formation (both active and inactive) and characteristic changes in the gland of hyperplasia, cystic degeneration, hemorrhage, colloid-filled follicles, fibrosis, and calcification. Severe iodine deficiency is associated with congenital hypothyroidism and cretinism. An estimated 12 million people worldwide suffer from some degree of mental impairment caused by iodine deficiency.

Although dietary goitrogens such as thiocyanate occur in cassava and vegetables of the brassica family, they are unlikely to produce a clinically significant goiter in the absence of iodine deficiency.

Prevention and Treatment

Prevention of simple endemic goiter requires the addition of iodine to the diet, commonly achieved by iodizing table salt. Oral or intramuscular administration of iodized oil is an appropriate alternative, especially in developing countries and areas where salt is not often consumed in the diet.

Diffuse, hyperplastic goiter at a prenodular stage can often regress significantly with the administration of thyroxine (0.1–0.15 mg daily) continued over several years. Thyroidectomy may be indicated for pressure symptoms unresponsive to medical treatment, for concern of malignancy, and occasionally for cosmetic reasons.

Sporadic Nontoxic Goiter

Sporadic, nontoxic goiter may be diffuse or nodular, occurs in iodine-sufficient regions, and is due to environmental and/or genetic factors.

Environmental: Anti-thyroid drugs such as carbimazole act at various sites within the thyroid gland to reduce thyroid hormone synthesis and may lead to goiter formation. In rare cases, excess iodine may cause goiter and hyperthyroidism (Jodbasedow phenomenon) or even hypothyroidism.

Genetic factors: An inherited deficiency of one or more of the enzymes responsible for the synthesis and secretion of thyroid hormone may result in a sporadic, dyshormonogenetic goiter. A deficiency in thyroid peroxidase, the enzyme responsible for organification of trapped iodides, results in Pendred's syndrome, characterized by congenital deafness and goiter in adolescence, and progression to multinodular thyroid. In severe forms, dyshormonogenesis will cause hypothyroidism and cretinism. Treatment is oral thyroxine, with thyroidectomy reserved for enlarging goiters causing pressure symptoms or cosmetic effects.

Thyroid Nodules

Many patients with nontoxic goiter describe the awareness of a swelling in the neck, but many are completely asymptomatic with the goiter detected during a routine physical examination for an unrelated condition. Sudden, painful swelling in the thyroid is likely to result from hemorrhage into a preexisting benign, colloid nodule. This condition usually resolves spontaneously in a few weeks without intervention, although aspiration can be helpful to relieve symptoms. Most nodular goiters and even malignant nodules may grow slowly for many years before a diagnosis is made. Rapid growth of an existing nodule with discomfort radiating into the face and jaw is suggestive of a poorly differentiated or anaplastic carcinoma, especially in the elderly.

In the USA, for instance, the prevalence of palpable thyroid nodules among individuals aged 30–59 years is about 4%. In autopsy series, the prevalence of thyroid nodules is as high as 50%. The majority of such nodules are less than 1 cm, benign, and include colloid lesions, follicular adenoma, nodular thyroiditis, and degenerative cysts.

When the lesion is solitary, the crucial clinical management issue is one of distinguishing between benign and malignant disease. The incidence of malignancy in a solitary thyroid nodule is approximately 10%, but is increased in men or when the nodule is enlarging. Goiters are more common in women than men. New nodules in children or the elderly must be regarded with high suspicion, because 50% of solitary nodules in children under 14 years of age are malignant.

Patients with a family history of thyroid cancer or other endocrine disease are more likely to have a malignant thyroid nodule. These syndromes include Multiple Endocrine Neoplasia types IIa and IIb (MEN IIa, MEN IIb) and non-MEN familial medullary thyroid cancer (FMTC).

Environmental and geographic factors are also relevant. Papillary thyroid cancer has an increased incidence in iodine-rich regions such as Iceland, whereas the incidence of follicular cancer is increased in endemic goiterous areas. Irradiation of the thyroid gland may induce thyroid malignancy, particularly papillary carcinoma. This relationship between thyroid carcinoma and a history of head and neck irradiation in children was first studied in 1950 and defined more precisely by DeGroot and Paloyan in 1973. The lag time from radiation to detection of malignancy ranges from 6 to 35 years. Although irradiation also increases the incidence of benign thyroid nodules, the risk of malignancy in a solitary palpable nodule in these patients ranges from 20% to 50%. The Chernobyl nuclear accident has been an unfortunate recent reminder of the powerful tumor-inducing effects of radiation. High-dose external radiation to the neck for conditions such as Hodgkin's lymphoma may also increase the risk of thyroid malignancy.

The initial clinical evaluation includes examination of the patient and assessment of thyroid function. Although most patients with a solitary nodule will be euthyroid, a nodule in the hyperthyroid patient is almost certain to be benign. Inspection and palpation assess whether the thyroid gland is diffusely enlarged or nodular. If nodular, then a distinction should be made between a solitary nodule, a multinodular goiter, or a dominant nodule within a multinodular gland. Previously, it had been accepted that the risk of malignancy in a multinodular goiter is low (approximately 1%); however, recent publications suggest that the incidence may not be dissimilar to that seen in solitary nodules, especially in the presence of a dominant nodule.

In addition to evaluation for size and nodularity, movement on swallowing and deviation of the trachea should be assessed. The likelihood of malignancy is increased in a hard, fixed nodule; however, a very hard lesion may represent a benign, calcified colloid nodule. Occasionally, soft nodules may be malignant as seen in cystic papillary neoplasms and follicular lesions with associated hemorrhage. Cervical lymphadenopathy in the setting of a thyroid nodule is likely to indicate a malignant rather than benign pathology. Hoarseness of the voice is a notoriously unreliable clinical sign, but a proven laryngeal nerve palsy on the side of a palpable thyroid nodule is very concerning for malignancy. Rarely, pressure effects from a benign thyroid lesion can result in vocal cord paralysis.

After careful clinical examination, thyroid functional status should be assessed by measurement of TSH and T4. It should be remembered that the elderly patient with longstanding nodular goiter may have few of the classic signs of hyperthyroidism; they may even have a normal serum T4, but increased T3 levels, indicating T3 thyrotoxicosis. When suspected, a chest x-ray may be useful to evaluate for tracheal deviation or retrosternal tumoral extension (Fig. 1.1). Measurement of serum calcitonin has been recommended in nodular goiters to detect C cell disease, but this practice is expensive, of low yield, and the cost-effectiveness has not been accepted universally. Measurement of antithyroid peroxidase antibodies (TPO) and thyroglobulin antibodies facilitate the diagnosis of autoimmune thyroiditis.

Thyroid Imaging

Although ultrasonography is capable of identifying multiple cystic and nonpalpable thyroid nodules, it is rarely capable of distinguishing between benign and malignant disease. Ultrasonography can be useful for monitoring change in the size of a thyroid lesion and will facilitate FNA biopsy of a suspicious lesion, when indicated by change in size or the

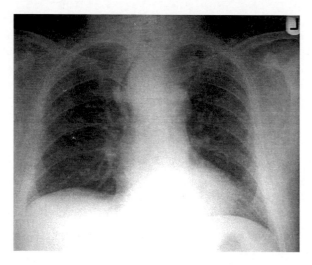

FIGURE I.I. Chest radiograph showing large retrosternal goiter causing tracheal deviation (Reprinted from Sadler and Wheeler (2001). Copyright 2001. With permission from Elsevier).

presence of a solid component in the wall of a cystic area. Ultrasonography should be employed selectively in the assessment of nontoxic thyroid disorders. Calcification within the thyroid is invariably coarse in benign disease and fine in some papillary and medullary cancers.

With the advent of more modern modalities (ultrasonography and FNA), radionuclide isotope scanning of the thyroid, either with ^{123}I or technetium pertechnetate 99mTc, has little value currently in the investigation of the patient with a thyroid nodule in the absence of associated thyrotoxicosis.

Needle Biopsy

FNA biopsy is the most valuable and diagnostically accurate investigation in thyroid nodular disease. The routine application of the technique in the patient with a clinical solitary nodule will allow many patients with benign disease to avoid an unnecessary thyroidectomy and facilitate the identification of those with a thyroid malignancy who require operative therapy. With the advent of image-guided needle biopsy of small, impalpable nodules, the identification of minute, occult thyroid cancers is not infrequent. Current opinion suggests that only a small minority of these histologic micro-carcinomas are relevant clinically, and the treatment of such lesions is somewhat controversial.

Treatment

A summary and scheme of management for patients with thyroid nodular disease is shown in Fig. 1.2. The majority of patients with benign goiter can be managed conservatively; however, operative intervention may be indicated for a significant group of patients with pressure and mechanical symptoms, including dyspnea, choking, and dysphagia. Retrosternal gland extension, especially if symptomatic or causing airway impairment as assessed by flow/volume/loop studies, is an indication for operative resection. Additionally, very large, disfiguring goiter may prompt operative intervention for cosmetic reasons. Each of the above indications is more likely to be found in multinodular rather than solitary nodule disease.

Operative treatment: For a solitary thyroid nodule, a unilateral total lobectomy with excision of the isthmus and pyramidal lobe is appropriate. This is a safe operation and permits a precise pathologic diagnosis, especially in those lesions which were suspicious or indeterminate on FNA. This approach obviates the need to reoperate at a later date for recurrent disease on the side of the original lesion, because any recurrent benign disease will inevitably be in the contralateral lobe.

When planning the extent of operation for multinodular goiter, there are more options, and the operative procedure may be based on intraoperative findings. Entirely unilateral disease is treated typically with unilateral thyroid lobectomy. Often there is asymmetrical nodularity, with one lobe considerably larger than the other. In these circumstances,

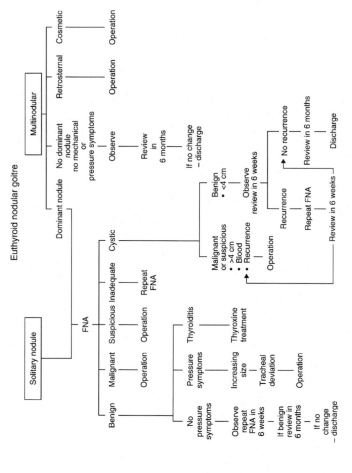

FIGURE I.2. Management scheme for patients with nodular thyroid disease.

unilateral total lobectomy with a subtotal procedure on the opposite side may be indicated. If there is bilateral enlargement and multinodularity, then a total thyroidectomy can be performed with a low risk to the recurrent laryngeal nerves and parathyroid glands provided the operation is performed by an experienced thyroid surgeon (Fig. 1.3).

Nonoperative therapy: Nonoperative therapeutic options include thyroxine therapy, which may decrease the size of a diffuse goiter in those suffering from iodine deficiency, or hypothyroidism. The benefits of thyroxine in nodular goiter are less apparent, and even when sufficient to suppress TSH, it is unlikely to improve pressure symptoms from an enlarged gland. In this setting, it is likely that other growth factors, such as EGF (epidermal growth factor) and IGF (insulin-like growth factor), may be influencing goiter size in addition to TSH. Radioiodine therapy can produce some shrinkage of the nontoxic goiter but is only likely to be indicated in the elderly or low-risk patient.

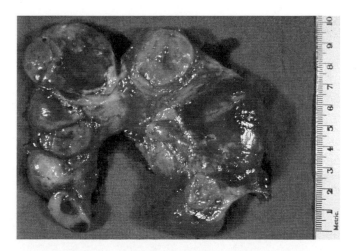

FIGURE 1.3. Benign multinodular goiter treated by total thyroidectomy (Reprinted from Maddox and Wheeler (2005). Copyright 2005. With permission from Elsevier).

Retrosternal Goiter

This is a particular, anatomic variant of a nodular goiter arising from downward growth of the thyroid into a substernal position. A thyroid which is palpable in the neck and has obvious extension posterior to the sternum is classified as substernal, whereas a gland entirely within the chest is termed intrathoracic. In some instances, retrosternal goiter may be asymptomatic and identified on chest x-ray obtained for other reasons. Usually, however, symptoms are common in these patients and include asthma, dysphagia, hoarseness of the voice, and other findings of airway compression. Vascular compression can also occur with perhaps the most dramatic example being superior vena cava obstruction. Pemberton's sign, in which there is distention of the external jugular and superficial neck veins on raising the arms above the head, is indicative of subclinical venous compression.

The retrosternal portion of such glands is not amenable to palpation or FNA for diagnostic purposes. Computed tomography (CT) (Fig. 1.4) and magnetic resonance imaging (MRI)

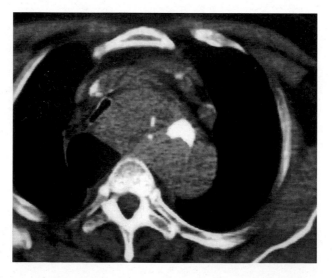

FIGURE 1.4. Computed tomography (CT) showing large intrathoracic goiter extending posterior to the trachea.

are extremely valuable investigations to define the true anatomic extent of the thyroid. Respiratory function tests with flow/volume/loop studies are also helpful.

The diagnosis of retrosternal goiter is typically an indication for operative intervention, in order to obtain a precise histologic diagnosis and prevent progressive airway obstruction or hemorrhage into a benign colloid lesion. Almost all retrosternal glands can be removed via a cervical surgical approach, with few (<1%) requiring a sternotomy.

Thyroiditis

Thyroiditis in an inflammatory disorder of the thyroid gland which may be focal or diffuse, acute, subacute, or chronic, and is often associated with thyroid dysfunction.

Acute Suppurative Thyroiditis

This condition, seen rarely in the developed world, is caused by a variety of bacterial or fungal organisms. The process produces an acute, painfully inflamed thyroid. Acute suppurative thyroiditis may result from infection of a persistent pyriform sinus or develop in the setting of immunosuppression. FNA for culture may identify the causative organism, frequently Staphylococcus, Streptococcus, and anaerobes, and thereby provide the opportunity for focused antimicrobial therapy. In the presence of abscess, aspiration or operative drainage may be required.

Subacute Thyroiditis (De Quervain's)

This painful condition is most likely of viral origin, and results in exquisite tenderness of one or both thyroid lobes, associated with fever and malaise. There is often a preceding history of sore throat or viral infection a week or two prior to the onset of thyroid symptoms. Some patients develop a more acute illness, with symptoms and signs of hyperthyroidism resulting from thyroid hormone release into the circulation from the inflamed, damaged thyroid. Serum concentrations of thyroid hormone are increased, but in marked contrast to the findings in Graves' disease, there is a low or absent uptake of radioactive iodine on scintigraphy. The sedimentation rate is increased invariably, and in approximately 20% of patients, there is an associated increase in thyroid antibody titers. Subacute thyroiditis is usually self-limiting with resolution of local symptoms and thyroid dysfunction. A few patients pass through a mild hypothyroid phase; however, full restoration to the euthyroid state occurs in more than 90% of patients. Local symptoms can be controlled with aspirin, but if the course of the disease is severe and prolonged, a trial of steroids may be appropriate. Transient hyperthyroidism does not require treatment with antithyroid drugs.

Autoimmune Thyroiditis (Hashimoto's)

Lymphocytic thyroiditis, a diffuse glandular inflammation, was first described by Hashimoto in 1912. Although thyroid gland enlargement is symmetrical classically, there may be nodularity and lobulation, which can make the distinction from simple multinodular goiter or even malignant disease difficult. Histologically, there is infiltration of the thyroid by lymphocytes and plasma cells, frequently secondary lymphoid nodules, and adjacent stromal fibrosis. This autoimmune disorder is characterized by an increase in serum thyroid antibodies, including antithyroglobulin and antithyroid peroxidase (TPO). A family history of other autoimmune disease is common, including pernicious anemia, gastritis, vitiligo, diabetes mellitus, Addison's disease, autoimmune liver disease, and thyrotoxicosis. The changes in the thyroid gland from lymphoid infiltration are destructive and have the potential to cause hypothyroidism with increased serum TSH levels, requiring treatment with thyroxine. By suppressing TSH secretion, administration of thyroxine causes shrinkage of the thyroid gland with optimal relief of local symptoms.

Operative intervention is indicated occasionally, but only when there are persistent symptoms from local pressure or cosmetic effects in spite of thyroxine medication.

Although rare, the incidence of thyroid lymphoma is increased several times in the presence of Hashimoto's thyroiditis. Such lymphomas are usually the non-Hodgkin's B-cell type, and the physician should be suspicious of this possibility when the thyroid enlarges rapidly or develops a firm, asymmetric nodular area. The diagnosis is confirmed by FNA or large bore needle biopsy.

Riedel's Thyroiditis

This condition, also known as invasive fibrous thyroiditis, is characterized by a dense, fibrous, inflammatory infiltrate throughout the gland, sometimes even extending through the capsule to involve adjacent structures. The process may result in a woody, hard, thyroid gland with fixation mimicking a locally advanced malignancy. A similar, sclerotic fibrosis may coexist in other sites, including sclerosing cholangitis, retroperitoneal, mediastinal, and retroorbital fibrosis. FNA biopsy is usually nondiagnostic, and an open incisional biopsy may be required. When there are significant symptoms, operative intervention may be required. A conventional thyroidectomy may be unsafe in this setting, and excision of the isthmus to free the compromised airway may be the most appropriate intervention. Options of medical treatment include steroids, which exhibit variable responses, or tamoxifen, which has demonstrated some benefit in the recent literature.

Post-partum Thyroiditis

This condition is characterized by an early toxic phase, usually with mild symptoms and transient dysfunction, and a later hypothyroid phase, sometimes requiring treatment with thyroxine. Long-term hypothyroidism may occur in up to 25% of patients.

Developmental Abnormalities of the Thyroid

Thyroglossal Cyst

Persistence of a portion of the thyroglossal duct results in a thyroglossal cyst, which is located typically in the midline (sometimes slightly lateral) just below the hyoid bone or above the thyroid cartilage. Less commonly, the cyst is located at a higher level above the hyoid bone. The classic diagnostic and clinical features are the presence of upward movement of the mass on swallowing, and especially with protrusion of the tongue due to attachment of the thyroglossal tract to the foramen cecum. These cysts are prone to infection and malignancy, typically papillary carcinomas may occur. The appropriate treatment is the Sistrunk procedure, which includes excision of the central portion of the hyoid bone. Infection or inadequate excision of a thyroglossal cyst may result in a thyroglossal fistula with an external cutaneous fistula opening low in the neck. Complete excision of the fistulous tract with the central hyoid is curative.

Lingual Thyroid

The thyroid gland may fail to descend and remain located in the posterior aspect of the tongue close to the foramen cecum. If large, the thyroid tissue can result in respiratory and swallowing difficulties and hemorrhage. Diagnosis is confirmed by radionuclide scanning. Treatment with thyroxine should result in shrinkage. Radioactive iodine is an alternative therapy, but operative excision is rarely necessary.

Ectopic Thyroid

When the descent of the thyroid gland is arrested during development, the gland can be located at any point along the line of the thyroglossal tract; in these circumstances, this ectopic thyroid may be the only thyroid tissue present (Fig. 1.5). Full thyroxine replacement will be required if operative excision is necessary.

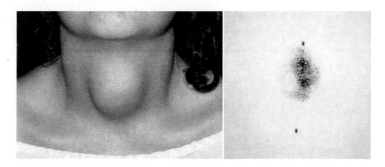

FIGURE 1.5. Ectopic undescended thyroid. Radioactive iodine scan shows functioning thyroid tissue at a site corresponding to the clinical mass without uptake in the expected location of the thyroid gland.

Selected Readings

Cheung PS-Y (2005) Medical and surgical treatment of endemic goiter. In: Clark OH, Duh Q-Y, Kebebew E (eds) Textbook of endocrine surgery, 2nd edn. Elsevier Saunders, Philadelphia, pp. 16–23

DeGroot LJ, Paloyan E (1973) Thyroid carcinoma and radiation: a Chicago endemic. JAMA 225:487–491

Franklyn JA, Daykin J, Young J, et al. (1993) Fine-needle aspiration cytology in diffuse or multinodular goiter compared with solitary thyroid nodules. BMJ 307:240

Harness JK, Thompson NW, Nishiyama RH (1971) Childhood thyroid carcinoma. Arch Surg 102:278–284

Maddox PR, Wheeler MH (2005) Approach to thyroid nodules. In: Clark OH, Duh Q-Y, Kebebew E (eds) Text-book of endocrine surgery, 2nd edn. Elsevier Saunders, Philadelphia, pp. 85–92

McCall A, Jarosz H, Lawrence AM, et al. (1986) The incidence of thyroid carcinoma in solitary cold nodules and in multinodular goiters. Surgery 100:1128

Sadler GP, Wheeler MH (2001) The thyroid gland. In: Farndon JR (ed) Endocrine surgery, 2nd edn. Elsevier Saunders, Philadelphia, pp. 39–87

Sirota DK, Segal RL (1979) Primary lymphomas of the thyroid gland. JAMA 242:1743–1746

Vander JB, Gaston EA, Dawber TR (1968) The significance of non toxic thyroid nodules: final report of a 15 year study of the incidence of thyroid malignancy. Ann Intern Med 69:537–540

Wheeler MH (1998) Total thyroidectomy for benign thyroid nodules. Lancet 351:1526–1527

2
Papillary Thyroid Cancer

Takashi Uruno and Orlo H. Clark

Pearls and Pitfalls

- Papillary thyroid cancer (PTC) accounts for 80% of all thyroid cancers and is the most rapidly increasing cancer in women in the United States.
- Latent thyroid cancer is present in 6.2–36% of thyroid glands at autopsy.
- Neck ultrasound evaluates the thyroid gland for suspicious nodules, as well as for thyroid cancer metastasis in cervical lymph nodes.
- Fine needle aspiration biopsy cytology (FNAC) under ultrasound guidance accurately diagnoses papillary, medullary, and anaplastic thyroid cancer and/or lymph node involvement.
- A total or near-total thyroidectomy is indicated for most patients with clinical thyroid cancer greater than 1 cm in size.
- Central neck and/or lateral neck dissection is indicated for clinically or scan-positive abnormal lymph nodes.
- A nonoperative approach is being done in Japan for patients with isolated micro PTC(≤1 cm) by FNAC without nodal involvement, in whom the tumor is not adjacent to the recurrent laryngeal nerve or trachea.

K.I. Bland et al. (eds.), *Endocrine Surgery*,
DOI: 10.1007/978-1-84996-447-0_2,
© Springer-Verlag London Limited 2011

- Regional lymph node recurrence develops in 5–20% of patients after thyroidectomy and appears to be lower after post thyroidectomy ablative treatment with ^{131}I and TSH suppressive therapy or with ipsilateral lymph node dissection.
- The mortality rate from PTC is primarily influenced by stage of disease and patient age.

Introduction

Thyroid cancer is the most common endocrine malignancy with approximately 30,000 new cases and 1,500 deaths estimated in 2006 year in the United States. It is the most rapidly increasing cancer and accounts for 3% of all cancers in woman. There are about 300,000 survivors of thyroid cancer in the USA. Papillary thyroid cancer (PTC) is the most common histological type of thyroid cancer, and accounts for approximately 80% of these tumors. Luckily, when PTC is well differentiated, it is the least aggressive type of thyroid cancer. PTC is more common in high-iodine intake countries or regions such as Iceland, Hawaii, and Japan; thus, PTC accounts for 90% of thyroid malignancies in Japan. Somatic BRAF point mutations are found in about 40% of PTC, and RET/PTC rearrangements are found in about 25%. Other mutations involved with thyroid cancer include TRK, MET and RAS. The ret/PTC oncogene is associated with pediatric PTC, radiation exposure and PTC microcarcinomas. BRAF mutations are found not only in well-differentiated PTCs, but also in poorly and undifferentiated thyroid cancers and are associated with a poorer outcome. Somatic p53 mutations are rare I well-differentiated thyroid cancers, but are common in anaplastic thyroid cancers.

Preoperative Diagnosis

A history should be taken regarding focal symptoms such as hoarseness, change in voice, dysphasia, or pain, and a history of exposure to low-dose therapeutic radiation or family history of thyroid cancer. Physical examination is important to identify the thyroid nodule or nodules and possible cervical lymphadenopathy. Ultrasonography combined with FNAC is the most important test for identifying and diagnosing thyroid cancer within the thyroid gland or in cervical lymph nodes. PTC can usually be diagnosed accurately by FNAC because of characteristic and clearly recognizable nuclear features. With an experienced cytologist, there is nearly 100% reliability.

Thyroglobulin measurement in fine needle aspiration biopsy washout is also a sensitive technique for diagnosing metastatic PTC in lymph nodes.

Treatment Option

Surgery

We believe that for most patients with thyroid cancer, including PTC, the initial surgical procedure should be a total or near-total thyroidectomy. Thyroid lobectomy, however, may be sufficient treatment for small, solitary, low-risk patients with PTCs in the absence of local invasion, cervical lymph node metastases, or distant metastasis. A routine ipsilateral central neck dissection (level VI) is recommended for patients with enlarged lymph nodes by ultrasonography, or when identified preoperatively or by physical examination at operation (Fig. 2.1). Lateral neck (compartments II–IV) and sometimes posterior triangle (V) dissection should be considered for patients in whom nodal disease is clinically evident, is identified on preoperative ultrasound, or at the time of surgery (Fig. 2.1). The value of prophylactic lateral node dissection is still controversial and is generally not recommended in the United States.

Complications after thyroidectomy include: bleeding, recurrent laryngeal nerve or external branch of the superior laryngeal nerve dysfunction, hypoparathyroidism, infection, neck edema, seroma, and keloid formation. Injury to the

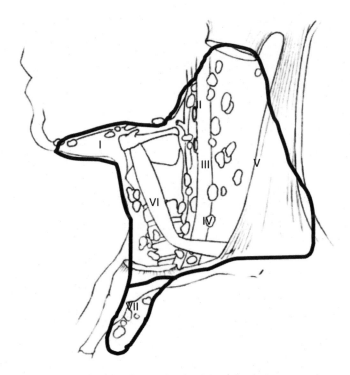

FIGURE 2.1. Cervical and mediastinal lymph node compartments. Level I – submental and submandibular nodes, Level II – upper internal jugular chain nodes, Level III – middle internal jugular chain nodes, Level IV – lower internal jugular chain nodes, Level V – spinal accessory and transverse cervical nodes, Level VI – tracheoesophageal groove nodes and perithyroidal nodes, and Level VII – infraclavicular and upper anterior mediastinal nodes (thymic) (Reprinted from Kebebew et al., 2003. Copyright 2003. With permission from Elsevier).

recurrent laryngeal nerve or hypoparathyroidism are frequent reasons for patient dissatisfaction. On rare occasions (0.63%), the right inferior laryngeal nerve does not recur but is nonrecurrent, whereas on the left side, this anomaly only occurs in patients with a right aortic arch with sinus inversus viscerum (0.04%). Nonrecurrence of the right inferior laryngeal nerve results from a vascular anomaly (an absent innominate artery, with an aberrant subclavian artery). Some surgeons recommend direct laryngoscopy to assess vocal cord function for all the patients before thyroid surgery; it is certainly essential for all patients with any voice change or for those who have a previous history of neck surgery. Some patients have asymptomatic vocal cord dysfunction due to tumor invasion, but also rarely from idiopathic paralysis.

Thyroid carcinomas of 10 mm or less in maximum diameter are defined as microcarcinoma, according to the World Health Organization classification. Papillary microcarcinomas are usually slow growing and rarely adversely influence survival. They may, however, be associated with lymph node metastasis. Periodic and careful follow-up without operation for patients with solitary microcarcinomas that are not situated posterior in the gland adjacent to the trachea and recurrent laryngeal nerve, and without FNAC findings suggesting high-grade malignancy, and/or lymph nodes highly suspicious of metastases, has been reported in Japan and the results warrant careful examination.

The finding of latent thyroid cancer at autopsy (6.2–36%) suggests that some elderly patients can be observed without thyroidectomy. However, because PTC in elderly patients may be biologically aggressive, surgery is generally recommended, even for the elderly patients (≥70 years), if the patient's general status is judged able to tolerate the stress of anesthesia and surgery.

Surgical resection remains the treatment of choice even for patients with locally advanced PTC including those with invasion into the recurrent laryngeal nerve, trachea, jugular vein, esophagus and carotidartery. At operation, a functioning recurrent laryngeal nerve should be preserved and dissected from adjacent invasive cancer or nodes. A primary anastomosis of the recurrent laryngeal nerve, interposition of a free nerve grafting, and anastomosis of the ansa hypoglossal nerve to the recurrent laryngeal nerve can improve phonation (prolong maximum phonation time) in patients who need resection of a unilateral recurrent laryngeal nerve.

For local recurrence in the neck or superior mediastinum, re-operation should be considered, as it appears to provide long-term palliation for many patients. A systematic (compartment-based) neck dissection preserving all motor and usually sensory nerves, not a selective dissection ("berrypicking"), is recommended to reduce the development of another local recurrence.

Postoperative treatment with ^{131}I after total thyroidectomy appears to decrease the risk for recurrent locoregional disease and facilitates long-term surveillance. Post-treatment imaging is more sensitive and accurate than pre-ablative scanning. Radioiodine ablation is recommended for patients with Stage III and IV disease, all patients with Stage II disease who are ≥45 years, most patients with Stage II disease who are <45 years, and selected patients with Stage I disease, especially those with multifocal disease, nodal metastases, extrathyroidal or vascular invasion, and/or more aggressive histological variations.

Patients with pulmonary micrometastases, which are detected only by diagnostic whole-body radioiodine scans and not observed on chest X-ray, should be treated with radioiodine therapy. These patients have excellent outcome. Radioiodine-avid pulmonary macronodular metastases and bone metastases should also be treated with radioiodine therapy, but complete remission is less common in these patients and survival remains poor.[5] For focal bone metastasis, resection followed by ^{131}I ablation or external radiation is indicated. Unfortunately, about 25% of patients with papillary thyroid cancer fail to have uptake of radioiodine.

TSH Suppressive Therapy

Suppression of TSH, using superphysiologic doses of LT_4, is frequently used to treat patients with differentiated thyroid cancer. TSH suppression to below 0.05 mU/l or 0.1 mU/l is recommended for high-risk patients, and at about 0.1 mU/l for low- to moderate-risk patients although the latter treatment is more controversial.

Other Treatment (External Radiation, Chemotherapy, Etc.)

The use of external beam irradiation should be considered in patients over age 45 with invasive papillary thyroid cancers that cannot be completely resected by an experienced thyroid surgeon. It is also indicated for patients who recur after re-resection in whom further surgery or radioactive iodine is unlikely to be effective. Doxorubicin (Adriamycin) has been used as a radiation sensitizer. There, unfortunately, is little data to support the use of adjunctive chemotherapy in the management of differentiated thyroid cancer. An experienced radiation therapist is important in order to decrease the risk of complications, especially injury to the spinal cord.

Follow-Up

Measurement of basal and TSH stimulated serum thyroglobulin levels is an important modality to monitor patients for residual papillary thyroid cancer (Table 2.1). Serum thyroglobulin should be measured every 6–12 months, and thyroglobulin antibodies should be quantitatively assessed with every measurement of serum thyroglobulin during follow-up of patients after total or near-total thyroidectomy. When

TABLE 2.1. Follow-up for patients with papillary thyroid cancer.

1. Serum thyroglobulin (basal and stimulated)[a]

2. Ultrasonography of neck

3. ^{131}I scan and ablative dose for all moderate- or high-risk patients, and those with an increased thyroglobulin or suspicious nodes

4. Fine needle aspiration cytology of suspicious nodule by ultrasound

5. Other scans (PET/MRI/CT) for thyroglobulin positive, radioiodine negative patients

6. TSH suppression

[a]After total or near total thyroidectomy.

thyroglobulin antibodies are present, the serum thyroglobulin is often not useful for the early detection of recurrence. Some authors suggest that elevated serum thyroglobulin antibody levels may serve as a surrogate marker for the presence of persistent thyroid cancer.

Because the most common site for recurrent PTC is in cervical nodes, annual cervical ultrasonography by an experienced radiologist is useful for identifying recurrent disease. Anaplastic transformation from a pre-existing differentiated cancer is an accepted process and occurs in about 1% of patients. Unfortunately, to date there is no good method for predicting which thyroid neoplasm will undergo anaplastic transformation.

Morphologic Variants, TNM Staging and Prognostic Factors

Some morphologic variants of PTC have been identified and are clinically used to determine the biological behavior of PTC (Table 2.2). A cribriform-morular variant (CMV) of PTC is a rare (0.16%) but unique histological type associated with familial polyposis and germline APC mutations. Patients with CMV should be screened for familial adenomatous polyposis-associated colon cancer, particularly when the patient has multiple tumors of the thyroid. The vast majority of patients with PTC and familial polyposis are women. Somatic RET/PTC mutations have been reported in about 80% of these thyroid cancers.

PTC is a fascinating tumor, as young patients do considerably better than older patients and women do better than men with comparably staged tumors (Table 2.3). Patients with locally invasive tumors, distant metastases, or a family history of thyroid cancer have a poorer prognosis. Numerous scoring systems have been reported to predict prognosis (Table 2.4a, b, and c).

Approximately one-third of the patients who develop recurrent thyroid cancer die of their disease. These deaths

TABLE 2.2. Morphologic variants of papillary carcinoma: behavior compared with classical papillary carcinoma.

Morphologic variants	Clinical behavior compared with typical PTC
Diffuse sclerosing variant	More aggressive
Diffuse follicular variant	
Tall cell variant	Probably more aggressive
Trabecular variant	
Dedifferentiated variant	More aggressive
Encapsulated variant	Better prognosis
Papillary microcarcinoma	
Follicular variant	Similar prognosis
Solid variant	
Oxyphil cell variant	
Variant with exuberant nodular fascitis-like stroma	Probably more aggressive
Macrofollicular variant	
Warthin tumor-like variant	
Cribriform-morular variant	
Variant with lipomatous stroma	

occur, although the presence of recurrence in regional lymph node probably has the least adverse effect on survival. These patients unfortunately present with diffusely metastatic disease to lung and bone sites. In spite of a higher *local* recurrence rate, patients with PTC have a favorable prognosis, whose 10-year relative survival rate is 98% compared with a population-based patient series. Unfortunately, patients continue to die from PTC up to 40 years after initial treatment.

New therapies are becoming available with anti-vascular endothelial growth factor (VEGF), anti-epidermal growth factor, and fibroblast growth factor, as well as an anti-tyrosine kinase activator (TKA). And other modulators of growth or apoptosis such as retinoids and peroxisome proliferator

TABLE 2.3. TNM classification system for differentiated thyroid carcinoma (American Joint Committee on Cancer, 2002).

Definition	
T1	Tumor diameter 2 cm or smaller
T2	Primary tumor diameter >2–4 cm
T3	Primary tumor diameter >4 cm limited to the thyroid or with minimal extrathyroidal extension
T4a	Tumor of any size extending beyond the thyroid capsule to invade subcutaneous soft tissues, larynx, trachea, esophagus, or recurrent laryngeal nerve
T4b	Tumor invades prevertebral fascia or encases carotid artery or mediastinal vessels
TX	Primary tumor size unknown, but without extrathyroidal invasion
N0	No metastatic nodes
N1a	Metastases to level VI (pretracheal, paratracheal, and prelaryngeal/Delphian lymph nodes)
N1b	Metastasis to unilateral, bilateral, contralateral cervical or superior mediastinal mode metastases
NX	Nodes not assessed at surgery
M0	No distant metastases
M1	Distant metastases
MX	Distant metastases not assessed

Stages	Patient < 45 years	Patient aged 45 years or older
Stage I	Any T, any N, M0	T1, N0, M0
Stage II	Any T, any N, M1	T2, N0, M0
Stage III		T3, N0, M0
		T1, N1a, M0
		T2, N1a, M0
		T3, N1a, M0

TABLE 2.3.(continued).

Stages	Patient < 45 years	Patient aged 45 years or older
Stage IVA		T4a, N0, M0
		T4a, N1a, M0
		T1, N1b, M0
		T2, N1b, M0
		T3, N1b, M0
		T4a, N1b, M0
Stage IVB		T4b, any N, M0
Stage IVC		Any t, any N, M1

TABLE 2.4a. AGES scoring system (Data from Hay et al., 1987. Reprinted from Treseler, 1997. Copyright 1997. With permission from Elsevier).

0.05 X age in years (if ≥40)	
+1	If tumor grade 2 (Broder's classification)
+2	If tumor grade 3 or 4 (Broder's classification)
+1	If extrathyroidal invasion by primary tumor
+3	If distant metastases
+0.2 X	Tumor size in centimeters
	= Total score (≥4 deemed high risk)

TABLE 2.4b. AMES risk groups (Data from Cady et al., 1998. Reprinted from Treseler, 1997. Copyright 1997. With permission from Elsevier).

Low risk

A. All younger patients (men ≤40, women ≤50) without distant metastases

B. All older patients with

  1. Intrathyroidal PTC, or FTC with minor tumor capsular invasion

  2. Primary tumor < 5cm

  3. No distant metastases

(*continued*)

TABLE 2.4b. (continued).

High risk
A. All patients with distant metastases
B. All older patients with
1. Extrathyroidal PTC, or FTC with major tumor capsular invasion
2. Primary tumor size ≥5 cm

PTC: papillary thyroid cancer; FTC: follicular thyroid cancer.

TABLE 2.4.c. MACIS scoring system (Data from Hay et al., 1993. Reprinted from Treseler, 1997. Copyright 1997. With permission from Elsevier).

+ 0.3 × Tumor size in cm
+ 1.0 If tumor incompletely excised
+ 1.0 If extrathyroidal invasion present
+ 3.0 If distant metastases present
= Total score (no definition high grade; four prognostic groups)

activated receptor γ (PPAR γ) activators are already being used in clinical trials. In the future, these new therapies with or without gene therapy will probably become effective treatments for patients with PTCs who fail conventional therapy.

Selected Readings

American Joint Committee on Cancer (2002) AJCC Cancer Staging Manual, 6th edn. Springer-Verlag, New York, www.springeronline.com

Cady B, et al. (1998) An expanded view of risk-group definition in differentiated thyroid carcinoma. Surgery 104:947–953

Caron NR, Clark OH (2004) Well differentiated thyroid cancer. Scand J Surg 93:261–271

Chan J (2000) Tumors of the thyroid and parathyroid glands. In: Fletcher CDM (ed) Diagnostic histopathology of tumors, 2nd edn. Churchill Livingstone, London

Cooper DS, Doherty GM, Haugen BR, et al. (2006) Management guidelines for patients with thyroid nodules and differentiated thyroid cancer. Thyroid 16:1–33

Gilliland FD, Hunt WC, Morris DM, Key CR (1997) Prognostic factors for thyroid carcinoma. A population-based study of 15,698 cases from the Surveillance, Epidemiology and End Results (SEER) program 1973–1991. Cancer 79:564–573

Hay ID, et al. (1987) Ipsilateral lobectomy versus bilateral lobar resection in papillary thyroid carcinoma: a retrospective analysis of surgical outcome using a novel prognostic scoring system. Surgery 102:1088–1095

Hay ID, et al. (1989) Predicting outcome in papillary thyroid carcinoma: development of a reliable prognostic scoring system in a cohort of 1779 patients surgically treated at one institution during 1940 through 1989. Surgery 114:1050–1058

Ito Y, Uruno T, Nakano K, et al. (2003) An observation trial without surgical treatment in patients with papillary microcarcinoma of the thyroid. Thyroid 13:381–387

Kebebew E, et al. (2003) Locally advanced differentiated thyroid cancer. Surg Oncol 12:91–99

Miyauchi A, Matsusaka K, Kihara M, et al. (1998) The role of ansa-to-recurrent-laryngeal nerve anastomosis in operations for thyroid cancer. Eur J Surg 164(12):927–933

Pacini F, Ladenson PW, Schlumberger M, et al. (2006) Radioiodine ablation of thyroid remnants after preparation with recombinant human thyrotropin in differentiated thyroid carcinoma: results of an international, randomized, controlled study. J Clin Endocrinol Metab 91:926–932

Pujol P, Daures JP, Nsakala N, Baldet L, Bringer J, Jaffiol C (1996) Degree of thyrotropin suppression as a prognostic determinant in differentiated thyroid cancer. J Clin Endocrinol Metab 81:4318–4323

Tomoda C, Miyauchi A, Uruno T, et al. (2004) Cribriform-morular variant of papillary thyroid carcinoma: clue to early detection of familial adenomatous polyposis-associated colon cancer. World J Surg 28(9):886–889

Treseler PA (1997) Prognostic factors in thyroid carcinoma. Surg Oncol Clin North Am 6:555–598

Uruno T, Miyauchi A, Shimizu K, et al. (2005) Favorable surgical results in 433 elderly patients with papillary thyroid cancer. World J Surg 29:1497–1501; discussion 502–503

Uruno T, Miyauchi A, Shimizu K, et al. (2004) Prognosis after reoperation for local recurrence of papillary thyroid carcinoma. Surg Today 34:891–895

Uruno T, Miyauchi A, Shimizu K, et al. (2005) Usefulness of thyroglobulin measurement in fine-needle aspiration biopsy specimens for
  diagnosing cervical lymph node metastasis in patients with papillary
  thyroid cancer. World J Surg 29:483–485
Wada N, Duh QY, Sugino K, et al. (2003) Lymph node metastasis from
  259 papillary thyroid microcarcinomas: frequency, pattern of occurrence and recurrence, and optimal strategy for neck dissection. Ann
  Surg 237:399–407
Wang HH (2006) Reporting thyroid fine-needle aspiration: literature
  review and a proposal. Diagn Cytopathol 34:67–76

3

Follicular, Hürthle Cell, and Anaplastic Thyroid Cancers

Chung-Yau Lo

Pearls and Pitfalls

- Follicular thyroid carcinoma (FTC) is a histologic subtype of well-differentiated thyroid carcinoma with distinct clinicopathologic features, biologic behavior, and prognosis.
- FTC cannot be diagnosed reliably by fine needle aspiration cytology or intraoperative frozen section examination. Diagnosis of follicular cancer (versus follicular adenoma) depends upon histologic evidence of unequivocal capsular and/or vascular invasion and usually requires tissue, not just cytology.
- FTC is categorized into histologic subtypes with implications for prognosis and management.
- Unilateral lobectomy is considered generally adequate for minimally invasive small (<2 cm) encapsulated FTC.
- Total thyroidectomy followed by radioiodine ablation is indicated for widely invasive FTC. The need for total thyroidectomy for angioinvasive FTC is controversial.
- Hürthle cell carcinoma is a more aggressive histologic variant of FTC because of its advanced presentation, propensity to metastasize, and decreased affinity for radioiodine.
- Anaplastic thyroid carcinoma, the most aggressive type of thyroid malignancy, presents usually as locally advanced disease with frequent distant metastases and is almost universally lethal; treatment is frequently palliative.

K.I. Bland et al. (eds.), *Endocrine Surgery*,
DOI: 10.1007/978-1-84996-447-0_3,
© Springer-Verlag London Limited 2011

- Operative resection followed by chemoirradiation for anaplastic thyroid carcinoma can be potentially curative, while preoperative hyperfractionated chemo-irradiation can palliate selected patients with locally advanced anaplastic lesions surrounding the trachea, often without the need of tracheostomy.

Follicular Thyroid Carcinoma

Follicular thyroid carcinoma (FTC) is a relatively rare form of thyroid cancer which accounts for 10–30% of well-differentiated thyroid carcinomas. FTC is more prevalent in areas with iodine-deficiency and endemic goiters; this prevalence may be attributed to the effect of thyroid-stimulating hormone. Iodine supplementation correlates with decreased incidence of FTC. Despite the fact that papillary and follicular thyroid carcinomas are classified collectively as well-differentiated thyroid cancers, they have distinct and different clinicopathologic features, biologic behavior, and clinical outcomes. FTC is considered generally to be a more aggressive neoplasm than papillary thyroid carcinoma and is associated with a worse prognosis. Patients with FTC present more often with distant metastases and more advanced stage disease. Nevertheless, patients with FTC should have a prognosis similar to those with PTC when they are matched for age and stage.

Clinical presentation: FTC is about 3–5 times more common in women than men. Patients present typically with a solitary thyroid nodule in the fourth or fifth decade of life. The incidence of lymph node metastases is much less than that of papillary thyroid cancer and is usually <10%. Conversely, hematogenous metastases are more common, and distant metastasis may be the first sign of the disease in 10–15% of patients with FTC. Metastases occur commonly in the lungs and bones, and particularly in the skull, manubrium, vertebral column, and long bones. Patients may present with an expanding sternal or skull mass, impending pathologic fracture of a long bone, or neurologic deficits secondary to spinal cord compression from vertebral metastases (Fig. 3.1). In contrast,

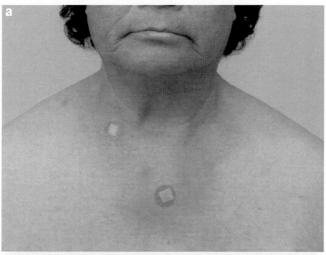

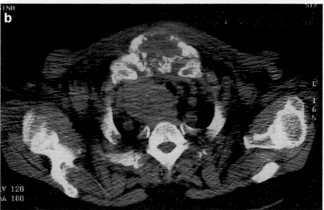

FIGURE 3.1. Widely invasive follicular thyroid carcinoma presenting with sternal metastases and right thyroid mass on (**a**) computed tomography and (**b**) clinical photos.

evidence of gross local invasion, which is an equivocal sign of malignancy, is encountered only infrequently. In the absence of either local invasion and/or distant metastases, the clinical diagnosis of FTC is difficult, and histologic examination of the entire surgical resection is imperative.

Diagnosis

Imaging studies are generally not helpful in establishing a definitive diagnosis of FTC. Ultrasonography can define several important characteristics of the nodule, such as size, echogenicity, and presence of capsule irregularity, tissue invasion, microcalcification, and hypervascularity. Ultrasonography can also detect additional nodules, assess for suspicious lymph nodes, and guide fine needle aspiration (FNA) cytology. Serum tests for thyroid function are generally within normal limits. FNA cytology is indicated for a solitary nodule or a dominant nodule in a multinodular gland, but the role of FNA cytology in the diagnosis of FTC remains unclear. FNA cytology for FTC is reported as "follicular neoplasm" or "follicular lesion," and such results are considered to be suspicious or atypical. Follicular neoplasm on FNA cytology represents a heterogeneous group of lesions, including benign follicular or adenomatous nodular hyperplasia, follicular adenoma, follicular carcinoma, and the follicular variant of papillary carcinoma. The overall incidence of malignancy for solitary thyroid nodules showing "follicular neoplasm" on FNA cytology ranges from 20% to 30%. Therefore, all patients with an FNA cytology report of "follicular neoplasm" probably require thyroidectomy.

Radioscintigraphy can be considered for patients with indeterminate cytology. In the presence of uptake (a functioning or warm nodule), the risk of malignancy is decreased substantially. In contrast, however, the majority of these nodules are nonfunctioning, cold lesions, and the diagnosis of malignancy cannot be confirmed or excluded by scintigraphy alone. In the presence of biochemical hyperthyroidism or clinical suspicion of a toxic adenoma, radioscintigraphy is indicated to assess the functional status of the nodule in correlation with malignant potential and to confirm the diagnosis of a toxic adenoma (Fig. 3.2).

In the absence of definitive features of local invasion or distant metastases, the diagnosis of malignancy in FTC requires identification of vascular or capsular invasion on

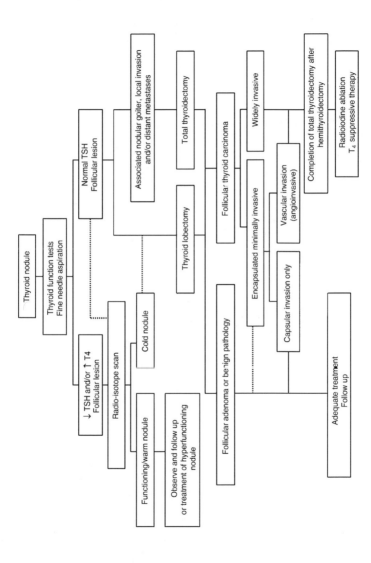

FIGURE 3.2. Staging/treatment algorithm for patients with thyroid nodule and a diagnosis of follicular neoplasm on fine needle aspiration cytology.

histologic examination. Therefore, the majority of patients with follicular neoplasm diagnosed on cytology require operative resection for definitive diagnosis. For patients with distant metastases, the diagnosis can be established by histologic examination of the biopsy from the distant metastases and confirmed by positive immunohistochemical staining with thyroglobulin.

Histologic Subtypes of FTC

Histomorphologic criteria have been utilized to differentiate FTC from follicular adenoma and to define the type and extent of invasion. Apart from classifying well-differentiated thyroid malignancies as extrathyroidal based on thyroid capsular extension, FTC is more commonly classified as either "minimally invasive encapsulated" or "widely invasive"; these two entities have a distinctly different biologic behavior and prognosis. Minimally invasive, encapsulated FTC resembles follicular adenoma grossly, and the diagnosis can only be made based on identification of full-thickness capsular penetration and/or vascular invasion by careful histologic examination with numerous serial tissue blocks (Fig. 3.3). In contrast to the minimally invasive type, widely invasive FTC comprises diffusely infiltrating, non-encapsulated or partly encapsulated neoplasms with extensive infiltration of surrounding non-neoplastic or vascular tissues. In addition, some investigators have suggested that minimally invasive, encapsulated FTC should be sub-classified into those neoplasms with capsular invasion alone (truly minimally invasive) and those with angioinvasion (moderately invasive or angioinvasive) because of the higher metastatic potential and a much poorer prognosis associated with vascular invasion (Fig. 3.4).

Molecular Basis and Its Role

Whether stringent histologic criteria should remain the gold standard for the diagnosis and sub-classification of FTC

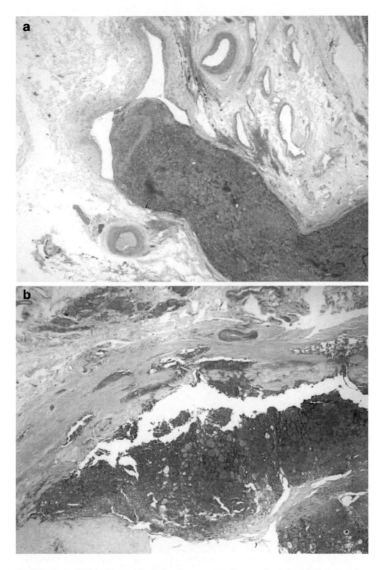

FIGURE 3.3. Histology of a lobectomy specimen showing (**a**) unequivocal capsular and (**b**) vascular invasion in follicular thyroid carcinoma.

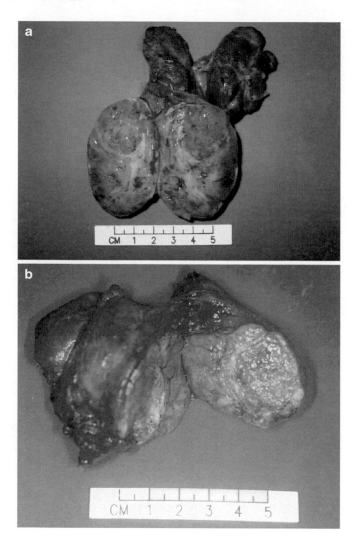

FIGURE 3.4. Characteristic gross appearance of (**a**) a well-encapsulated follicular thyroid neoplasm and (**b**) a widely invasive follicular carcinoma.

remains controversial. Substantial intraobserver variability occurs in the assessment of follicular lesions. In addition, it remains unclear whether FTC arises from a pre-existing follicular adenoma and progresses sequentially from minimally to widely invasive cancer with the accumulation of genetic alterations. A variety of molecular markers appear promising in the diagnosis and genetic subclassification of follicular cancer. These molecular markers include RAS mutations, expression of 72-kd Type IV collagenase, telomerase, galactin III, COX 2, and PAX8/PPARγ, detection of chromosomal abnormalities and imbalances by comparative genomic hybridization, and identification of areas of loss of heterozygosity by gene mapping and gene profiling by cDNA microarray. These techniques offer potential insight into the natural history and prediction of the clinical course of the disease.

Treatment and Outcome

FTC is associated with a 10-year survival rate of 70–95%. Total thyroidectomy followed by radioiodine ablation is recommended for all patients with widely invasive FTC. Several variables, including older age, distant metastases at presentation, extrathyroidal invasion, nodal metastases, larger tumor size, marked vascular invasion, widely invasive histology, and postoperative locoregional disease, have been identified as independent prognostic factors for survival in multivariate analyses. The identification of these risk factors is important in facilitating the optimal management protocol for individual patients. In addition, commonly adopted risk group stratification, classification, staging, and prognostic scoring schemes for well-developed thyroid malignancies can be applied specifically to patients with FTC with similar prognostic accuracy. These risk-related groups may define a subset of patients in whom a more limited operative approach without the need for radioiodine treatment may be considered.

Despite its lack of prognostic significance, the differentiation of FTC into minimally invasive and widely invasive carcinomas is employed commonly for the identification of low-risk patients for a more conservative, overall surgical management. Encapsulated, minimally invasive FTC comprises approximately 40% (10–50%) of FTC and is associated with excellent prognosis; long-term recurrence rates are <5%. Although total thyroidectomy remains the procedure of choice for widely invasive FTC, unilateral lobectomy is accepted increasingly to be adequate treatment for minimally invasive, encapsulated FTC. In addition, FTC with capsular invasion alone behaves like a benign neoplasm, with no disease-specific mortality or distant metastases at 10-year follow-up, regardless of primary treatment. Some studies have suggested that minimally invasive FTC with vascular invasion should be distinguished from those with capsular invasion alone. Vascular invasion may be a better indication of malignancy because of the greater probability of recurrence and metastases in the presence of angioinvasion. The presence of vascular invasion alone increases the disease-specific mortality to 28% at 10 years, although in multivariate analysis, the presence of distant metastases proved to be the only independent prognostic factor for survival. Because of the potentially worse prognosis and aggressiveness of minimally invasive FTC with vascular invasion, angioinvasive FTC probably should be classified separately and should be managed more aggressively by total thyroidectomy followed by radioiodine ablation.

For the majority of patients without local invasion or distant metastases, the definitive diagnosis of FTC and its histologic subtype requires a careful histologic examination. In contrast to PTC, intraoperative frozen section analysis provides relevant information infrequently and often unreliably, rarely should modify the operative decision, and occasionally misguides intervention for patients with FTC requiring unilateral lobectomy. For patients with FTC who require total thyroidectomy but have undergone an initial lobectomy, completion total thyroidectomy by removal of the contralateral lobe should be performed preferably within 1 week after the initial operation to facilitate the operation and allow radioiodine therapy, detection of distant metastases, and monitoring of postoperative thyroglobulin. The use of total thyroidectomy and radioiodine therapy improves the survival of patients with widely invasive FTC, even for those patients with distant metastases or residual disease after incomplete excision.

Hürthle Cell Carcinoma

Hürthle cells, also known as oncocytic or oxyphilic cells, are characterized as large polygonal and eosinophilic cells with small pleomorphic, hyperchromatic, pyknotic central nuclei and distinct, fine granular, acidophilic cytoplasm, representing an abundance of mitochondria. To be considered as a Hürthle cell neoplasm, more than 75% of the tumor must consist of Hürthle cells. Hürthle cell carcinoma is classified as a variant of FTC by the World Health Organization and accounts for 20% of FTC. Hürthle cell carcinoma is a rare type of thyroid cancer, and only about 400 patients have been reported since 1935. Some investigators classify Hürthle cell carcinomas separately because of the distinct difference in molecular alterations, chromosomal rearrangements, and clinical features from FTC. The diagnosis of Hürthle cell carcinoma is identical to that of FTC and is based on the unequivocal histologic criteria of malignancy which includes the presence of capsular and/or vascular invasion.

Clinical Features and Diagnosis

Patients with Hürthle cell carcinoma present most frequently between the fifth and seventh decades of life, slightly older than for most other well-developed thyroid malignancies. Like other thyroid cancers, Hürthle cell carcinoma occurs more frequently in women. These neoplasms are remarkably similar to FTC on gross examination, but are more likely to present as advanced or aggressive diseases. Hürthle cell carcinoma is also more likely to be multifocal within the thyroid gland, have nodal metastases, and progress after low-dose radiation. Contralateral foci of tumor are reported in 40–70%

of Hürthle cell carcinoma, while lymph node metastases occur in 10–25% of patients.

In evaluating a thyroid nodule, although FNA cytology can readily distinguish Hürthle cell neoplasm from non-neoplastic lesions, it cannot differentiate Hürthle cell adenoma reliably from carcinoma. About 25% of these lesions ultimately prove to be malignant, but the prevalence ranges from 5% to 60%. The size of a Hürthle cell neoplasm has been shown to correlate with its malignant potential and its aggressiveness. Similar to follicular lesions, operative treatment is recommended for patients in whom FNA cytology demonstrates a Hürthle cell neoplasm.

Treatment and Outcome

Hürthle cell carcinoma has a high propensity for distant metastasis and a low affinity for radioiodine uptake, resulting in an overall worse prognosis than that of FTC; however, survival of patients is similar to that of FTC when matched for stage. Male sex, tumors > 4 cm, extrathyroidal extension, widely invasive carcinoma, nodal metastases, and overall stage are prognostic factors for poor survival, although the presence of distant metastases is usually the strongest predictor.

One-stage total or near-total thyroidectomy is indicated for Hürthle cell carcinoma provided a careful operative exploration detects obvious malignant disease in the presence of tumor invasion to adjacent structures and/or lymph node metastases. Similarly, this operative strategy can also be adopted in the presence of nodular, contralateral lobar disease, distant metastases, or a positive history of childhood head and neck irradiation. For patients with a single dominant nodule, operative management should consist of a unilateral lobectomy and isthmusectomy. Routine frozen section can be omitted because of its limitation in detecting capsular and/or vascular invasion similar to that for follicular neoplasm. Enlarged or suspicious lymph nodes in the central or lateral compartments should be excised; indeed, a prophylactic ipsilateral central nodal dissection is recommended frequently due to the increased incidence of nodal metastases and recurrence compared with FTC. A completion total thyroidectomy by contralateral lobectomy should be performed in patients after an initial hemithyroidectomy, except for those encapsulated, Hürthle cell cancers with capsular invasion only. Although fewer than 10% of these cancers take up radioiodine, any thyroid remnant after total or near-total thyroidectomy should be ablated with radiolabeled iodine[131] to eliminate all tissue at risk and to facilitate the use of serum thyroglobulin in surveillance for tumor recurrence.

In selected patients, recurrent disease can be treated surgically with either curative or palliative intent, frequently resulting in prolonged survival. Local excision with nodal dissection for recurrent cervical disease, and even operative resection for *isolated* bone metastases and lung metastasis, have been shown to be effective. All patients with Hürthle cell cancers should be given thyroid hormone suppression, because most of these neoplasms have thyrotropin receptors. External beam radiation may be considered for patients with unresectable disease for palliative purposes when there is no uptake of radioiodine.

Anaplastic Thyroid Carcinoma

Anaplastic or undifferentiated carcinoma of the thyroid gland, albeit rare, is considered one of the most lethal of human malignancies and carries a dismal prognosis. Although anaplastic thyroid cancer constitutes only 2–10% of thyroid cancers, it accounts for more than half of all the deaths related to thyroid cancer. Despite an overall increase in the number of well-differentiated thyroid malignancies, the relative incidence of anaplastic thyroid carcinoma appears to be declining in many communities, probably due to early detection and subsequent aggressive resection of thyroid neoplasms, iodine prophylaxis, and improvement in socioeconomic status.

The presence of concomitant, well-differentiated thyroid malignancies is a common finding reported in 24–89% of anaplastic thyroid cancers. The co-existence or histologic association supports the theory of stepwise de-differentiation or transformation of human thyroid carcinomas, from well-differentiated to poorly differentiated and undifferentiated neoplasms. The rate of transformation, however, is low and has been estimated at <1%. Anaplastic thyroid cancers and co-existing well-differentiated thyroid malignancies share a core of genetic loci with identical allelic imbalance. The anaplastic component shows accumulation of additional loci of allelic loss, consistent with the multistep carcinogenesis with acquired mutational damage.

Clinical Presentation

The peak incidence of anaplastic thyroid carcinomas occurs in the sixth to seventh decade of life; this neoplasm is exceedingly rare in patients younger than 40 years of age. Patients typically have a longstanding history of goiter and present with a rapidly enlarging, firm-to-hard neck mass fixed to underlying structures. Pressure symptoms are usually present. Hoarseness of voice may be due to an underlying recurrent laryngeal nerve palsy in 30% of patients. Anaplastic cancer invades the contiguous structures commonly, such as the trachea, larynx, esophagus, carotid vessels, and the overlying skin causing necrosis in up to 70% of patients. Tracheal compression and cord palsy can result in shortness of breath and airway obstruction (Fig. 3.5). Cervical nodal metastases are present in up to 40% of patients. Distant metastases involving the lung, bone, brain, liver, and adrenal glands occur in 50% of patients at presentation and in another 25% of patients during the course of the disease.

Diagnosis

Diagnosis is usually suspected on clinical grounds. FNA cytology can confirm the diagnosis of anaplastic thyroid carcinoma in 90% of patients, but must be differentiated from thyroid lymphoma, medullary thyroid carcinoma, and poorly

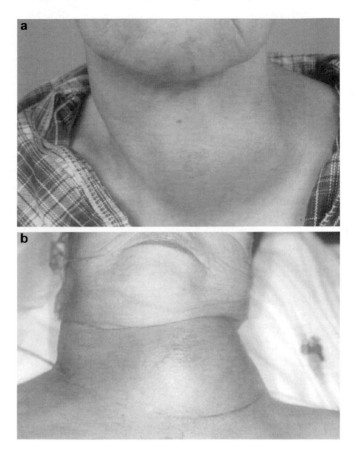

FIGURE 3.5. An elderly patient with a rapidly enlarging anaplastic thyroid carcinoma (**a**). The neoplasm grew rapidly within 4 weeks after presentation with evidence of skin involvement and airway obstruction (**b**).

differentiated thyroid carcinoma by immunophenotyping and other appropriate marker examinations. Core or open biopsy may be required in the setting of diagnostic uncertainty. The diagnosis can also be confirmed by biopsy of any detectable nodal or distant metastases or may be an incidental finding in patients undergoing thyroidectomy for well-differentiated thyroid malignancy. Patients diagnosed with anaplastic thyroid carcinoma should be managed expediently to avoid the eminent airway obstruction. The development of anaplastic thyroid carcinoma from an underlying well-differentiated thyroid malignancy may pose occasionally a diagnostic dilemma and impose a management challenge when FNA cytology fails to sample the anaplastic component. In contrast to the operative treatment for locally advanced well-differentiated thyroid malignancy, radical resection is avoided generally for anaplastic thyroid carcinoma. Despite aggressive resectional treatment, prognosis is invariably poor due to the frequent occurrence of distant metastases and the lack of effective adjuvant therapies. Hence, the operative treatment is largely palliative in nature, although on occasion, radical en-bloc resection should be entertained.

Treatment and Outcome

Anaplastic carcinoma of the thyroid gland is a very aggressive cancer and is almost invariably fatal, with the exception of incidentally detected focal or encapsulated lesions arising from malignant transformation of pre-existing, well-differentiated thyroid malignancy. Death is invariable in the majority of patients; the median survival is less than 6–12 months. Management of patients with anaplastic thyroid carcinoma is difficult because of the delayed and advanced clinical presentation, the frequent occurrence in elderly frail patients with a poor medical condition, the aggressiveness of tumors, and the relative lack of effective treatment options. Despite the frequent occurrence of distant metastases, the majority of patients die from complications of uncontrolled local cervical disease. Hence, achieving local control may improve short-term survival rates and obtain effective palliation.

The current operative approach seems to have evolved from palliative tracheostomy alone, to complete local resection for palliation or potential cure. Resectional ablation is adopted frequently in selected patients as the first-line treatment to remove or debulk the locally invasive and obstructing cancer. Radical en-bloc resection may be of value as a palliative measure to avoid future upper airway obstruction and is potentially curative when followed by postoperative chemoirradiation. This strategy, however, is not be feasible in the majority of poor risk patients, and aggressive resection should not be contemplated in the presence of distant metastases or locally advanced disease. Palliative tracheostomy is indicated for some patients during the course of the disease for impending airway obstruction rather than as a routine prophylactic measure.

Conventional chemotherapeutic agents do not prolong the survival of patients with anaplastic thyroid carcinoma. Doxorubicin is the drug used most frequently, but monotherapy has ≤20% response rate without complete response. Combination chemotherapeutic regimens with the addition of cisplatin, cyclophosphamide, or bleomycin marginally increase the clinical response rate, but newer agents such as paclitaxel as a single agent demonstrate an improved response rate of about 50%.

Radiotherapy alone does not alter the course of patients with anaplastic thyroid carcinoma. When combined with radiotherapy, thyroidectomy and chemotherapy can improve local control and radiosensitivity, respectively. Radiotherapy can be given either preoperatively to enhance resectability or postoperatively to improve local control. The delivery of radiotherapy with a hyperfractionating protocol and an accelerated dose schedule, combined with chemotherapy, can enhance its efficacy but must be balanced with its increased toxicity. Operative resection can be considered for responders. While no survival benefit has been documented, local control can be improved, and the need for tracheostomy or the occurrence of death secondary to airway obstruction may be avoided.

Although combination multimodality treatment improves outcome, the sequence of each treatment modality remains unclear, and there is no effective cure. Current investigations into an alternative therapeutic strategy include targeted molecular therapies. Inhibitors of epidermal growth factor and vascular endothelial growth factor, administration of adenoviral vectors containing the wild type tumor suppressor gene p53, bovine seminal ribonuclease, and vascular targeting agents such as combretastatin A4, alone or in combination with paclitaxel, have been shown to inhibit cellular proliferation and induce apoptosis in cell lines of anaplastic thyroid cancer in vitro, as well as to achieve control of tumor growth in xenograft models in nude mice. The development of these novel anticancer therapies will hopefully prove promising in the treatment of this uniformly fatal disease.

Selected Readings

Are C, Shaha AR (2006) Anaplastic thyroid carcinoma: biology, pathogenesis, prognostic factors and treatment approaches. Ann Surg Oncol 13:453–464

D'Avanzo A, Ituarte P, Treseler P, et al. (2004) Prognostic scoring systems in patients with follicular thyroid cancer: a comparison of different staging systems in predicting the patient outcome. Thyroid 14:453–458

Ghossein RA, Hiltzik DH, Carlson DL, et al. (2006) Prognostic factors of recurrence in encapsulated Hürthle cell carcinoma of thyroid gland. Cancer 106:1669–1676

Hunt JL, Tometsko M, LiVolsi VA, et al. (2003) Molecular evidence of anaplastic transformation in coexisting well-differentiated and anaplastic carcinomas of the thyroid. Am J Surg Pathol 27:1559–1564

Kebebew E, Greenspan FS, Clark OH, et al. (2005) Anaplastic thyroid carcinoma. Treatment outcome and prognostic factors. Cancer 103:1330–1335

Lo CY, Chan WF, Lam KY, et al. (2005) Follicular thyroid carcinoma: the role of histology and staging systems in predicting survival. Ann Surg 242:708–715

Lo CY, Lam KY, Wan KY (1999) Anaplastic carcinoma of the thyroid. Am J Surg 177:337–339

Stojadinovic A, Ghossein RA, Hoos A, et al. (2001) Hürthle cell carcinoma: a critical histopathologic appraisal. J Clin Oncol 19: 2616–2625

Thompson LDR, Wieneke JA, Paal E, et al. (2001) A clinico-pathologic study of minimally invasive follicular carcinoma of the thyroid gland with a review of the English literature. Cancer 91:505–524

4
Medullary Thyroid Carcinoma

Henning Dralle and Andreas Machens

Pearls and Pitfalls

- Medullary thyroid carcinoma, or C cell carcinoma, comes in a sporadic (75%) and a hereditary (25%) variant. Present in both conditions, C cell hyperplasia is a recognized intermediate stage in the progression from normal C cells to hereditary, but not sporadic medullary thyroid carcinoma.
- The presenting symptoms of medullary thyroid carcinoma mostly arise from primary tumor growth (60–80%) and cervical lymph node enlargement (20–40%). Occasionally, increased levels of calcitonin or carcinoembryonic antigen (CEA), protracted diarrhea, or the presence of gross distant metastases herald the disease.
- In multiple endocrine neoplasia type 2, hereditary medullary thyroid carcinoma usually (>90%) is the first neuroendocrine neoplasm to develop, followed by pheochromocytoma and primary hyperparathyroidism. Familial thyroid carcinoma (FMTC, or MTC-only) represents a less penetrant, late-onset variant within the MEN2 spectrum, rather than a tumor entity in its own right.
- Calcitonin is the principal secretory product of medullary thyroid carcinoma. Basal serum levels of calcitonin reflect overall tumor burden and may serve as a surrogate for tumor stage. Increased CEA serum levels indicate advanced tumor growth, lymph node involvement, and distant metastases.

K.I. Bland et al. (eds.), *Endocrine Surgery*,
DOI: 10.1007/978-1-84996-447-0_4,
© Springer-Verlag London Limited 2011

- The pentagastrin-triggered release of calcitonin from secretory vesicles into the bloodstream is essential for the diagnosis of occult medullary thyroid carcinoma. Unfortunately, pentagastrin stimulation may cause unpleasant side effects. The availability of this agent has become restricted in some countries.
- DNA-based RET analysis has become the gold standard for the diagnosis of hereditary C cell disease, enabling early identification of asymptomatic RET carriers. Because of the profound implications of a diagnosis of heredity, and because of the rarity of medullary thyroid carcinoma in the general population, every patient with medullary thyroid carcinoma should undergo DNA analysis. There is a marked genotype-phenotype correlation, not just with regard to the penetrance of the MEN 2 syndrome, i.e., the additional development of pheochromocytoma and primary hyperparathyroidism, but also with regard to the speed of progression from C cell hyperplasia to medullary thyroid carcinoma.
- In patients with medullary thyroid carcinoma, tumor stage at the time of surgery is the only significant indicator of survival. Altogether, 5-year survival rates approximate 80%, and 10-year survival is 65%. Long-term survival is excellent, despite low rates of postoperative calcitonin normalization (approximately 60% with node-negative cancers, and approximately 10% with node-positive cancers).
- Only second to undifferentiated thyroid carcinoma, medullary thyroid carcinoma is notorious for early spread to regional lymph nodes and distant organs.
- Because of their frequent involvement, the central lymph nodes of the neck should be removed at the initial operation along with the thyroid gland. When the central cervical lymph nodes are positive, the lateral cervical lymph nodes on the side of the primary thyroid tumor almost always are involved as well. Less often affected are the opposite lateral cervical and the mediastinal lymph nodes, but if so, this involvement is indicative of distant metastasis.

• Systemic disease may arise from thyroid microcarcinomas, i.e., tumors measuring 10 mm or less. In the absence of gross cervical metastases, increased calcitonin levels hint at the existence of minimal residual disease. In contrast to patients who have minimal residual disease, patients with gross metastases often develop progressive disease warranting additional systemic treatment.

Introduction

Making up 5–10% of all thyroid malignancies, medullary thyroid carcinoma, which originates from neural crest-derived parafollicular C cells, fundamentally differs in genetics and tumor biology from follicular cell-derived papillary, follicular, and undifferentiated thyroid carcinomas. Normal, hyperplastic, and neoplastic C cells secrete calcitonin, CEA, and other biogenic amines which may cause diarrhea. Loss of the capacity to secrete calcitonin is exceptional (<1%) and may indicate dedifferentiation in more advanced tumors. Unable to express the sodium/iodine symporter, C cells do not concentrate iodine, rendering radioiodine useless for the treatment of medullary thyroid carcinoma. As no other effective therapies exist, surgery remains the mainstay of therapy, especially for disease confined to the neck. In locally progressive unresectable disease, percutaneous radiation may be beneficial. Novel therapeutic modalities, such as immunotherapy targeted against somatostatin, gastrin, or CEA receptors, and tyrosine kinase inhibitors, are under development.

Sporadic C-Cell Hyperplasia and Medullary Thyroid Carcinoma

DNA-based RET analysis forms the cornerstone of disease management, enabling an early distinction between hereditary and sporadic medullary thyroid carcinoma. Additional life-long screening for pheochromocytoma and primary hyperparathyroidism is required in patients with hereditary, but not with sporadic tumors.

Considering the high prevalence of lymph node metastases from medullary thyroid microcarcinomas, all in all some 25% in tumors measuring ≤10 mm, early diagnosis through calcitonin screening is of paramount importance. Despite the low incidence of medullary thyroid carcinoma among patients with nodular goiter, there is a significant survival advantage for a symptomatic patient with occult C cell disease identified through calcitonin screening over symptomatic patients with overt medullary thyroid carcinoma.

It was only through the widespread adoption of biochemical screening that a new disease entity, sporadic C cell hyperplasia, emerged on the scene. Biochemical distinction between C cell disease and medullary microcarcinoma is a real challenge as calcitonin levels largely overlap between the conditions. With stimulated calcitonin levels below 100 pg/ml, medullary thyroid carcinoma is uncommon. Above that threshold, the risk of medullary thyroid carcinoma increases appreciably. When stimulated calcitonin levels exceed 500 pg/ml, medullary thyroid carcinoma is fairly common. Despite extensive research in this area, "neoplastic" C cell hyperplasia has remained elusive, casting doubt on the concept of a natural progression from sporadic C cell hyperplasia to sporadic medullary thyroid carcinoma. Of note, C cell hyperplasia also occurs in some 20% of patients with chronic lymphocytic thyroiditis and in some 30% of adults without identifiable thyroid disease on autopsy. Unlike hereditary C cell hyperplasia for hereditary medullary thyroid carcinoma, sporadic C cell hyperplasia cannot be regarded as a preneoplastic condition for medullary thyroid carcinoma in RET-negative patients.

For clinical purposes, the following algorithm has been devised (Fig. 4.1). Patients with biochemical evidence of C cell hyperplasia who have not had total thyroidectomy should undergo DNA-based RET analysis to exclude hereditary C cell disease.

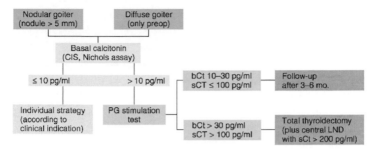

FIGURE 4.1. Routine calcitonin screening in nodular thyroid disease and indication for thyroidectomy. Notes: bCT: basal calcitonin; sCt: stimulated calcitonin; PG: pentagastrin; LND: lymph node dissection (Modified from Karges et al., 2004).

Clinical Presentation

When malignant thyroid nodules and lymph node metastases are the presenting symptoms, postoperative normalization of calcitonin levels is rarely (<20%) feasible. Because diarrhea and increased stool frequency are associated with advanced disease, these symptoms may portend a bleaker prognosis. Although the surgical consequences may not differ between local and systemic disease, additional imaging is generally recommended in suspected systemic disease for tumor staging. In the face of systemic disease, long-term survival may be acceptable or even excellent in most patients. All surgical efforts therefore should be directed at preventing disease-related local complications such as the invasion of adjacent structures, especially of the larynx, trachea, esophagus, or recurrent laryngeal nerves.

Medullary Thyroid Carcinoma as One Component of the MEN 2 Spectrum

Some 25 different hot-spot germline mutations have been identified in the RET protooncogene, all of which may cause hereditary medullary thyroid carcinoma. These point mutations have been found in almost all FMTC and MEN 2 families. The penetrance of hereditary C cell hyperplasia reaches almost 100%. Nevertheless, just 70% of all RET gene carriers develop overt medullary thyroid carcinomas by the age of 70 years. The time frame required for progression from C cell hyperplasia to medullary thyroid carcinoma was estimated at 2–5 years depending on the type of the RET mutation. Progression is faster in carriers of extracellular-domain RET mutations in codon 609, 611, 618, 620, 630, and 634, and slower in carriers of intracellular domain mutations in codon 768, 790, 791, 804, and 891.

The clinical presentation of hereditary medullary thyroid carcinoma does not differ from the manifestation of sporadic medullary thyroid carcinoma. Most RET carriers first develop medullary thyroid carcinomas, followed by pheochromocytoma and primary hyperparathyroidism. The penetrance of the various neuroendocrine neoplasms is dependent on the type of the RET mutation. Carriers of extracellular-domain mutations in codon 609, 611, 618, 620, 630, and 634 are more prone to develop pheochromocytomas and primary hyperparathyroidism and thus the full-blown MEN 2 syndrome than carriers of intracellular-domain mutations in codon 768, 790, 791, 804, and 891. As the progression of neuroendocrine tumors cannot be predicted individually, screening should also be instituted in the latter group of RET carriers.

Calcitonin and CEA as Tumor Markers of Medullary Thyroid Carcinoma

Unlike patients with medullary microcarcinoma, which is detectable through calcitonin stimulation only, almost all other patients with sporadic and hereditary medullary thyroid carcinoma feature increased basal calcitonin levels. Barring rare instances of hypercalcitoninemia produced by extrathyroidal neuroendocrine malignancies, increased basal calcitonin levels are the biochemical hallmark of medullary thyroid carcinoma. In contrast to calcitonin which is stored in secretory vesicles and released on stimulation, CEA as a membrane-bound protein is less susceptible to stimulation and therefore less suited for the diagnosis of occult disease. Sometimes, increased CEA serum levels are the sole evidence of occult medullary thyroid carcinoma.

The higher preoperative calcitonin and CEA levels, the worse the outcome. Preoperative basal calcitonin levels in excess of 500 pg/ml were found to best predict the failure of postoperative calcitonin to revert to normal, irrespective of heredity. These calcitonin levels were more important than the presence of lymph node metastases or surgical status (i.e., reoperation). When these calcitonin levels exceeded 3,000 pg/ml, patients with node-positive cancers no longer attained normalization of serum calcitonin despite extensive surgical intervention. With basal calcitonin levels as low as 10–40 pg/ml, lymph node metastases can be present. Extrathyroidal growth and distant metastases were noted with basal calcitonin levels as low as 150–400 pg/ml.

Postoperative calcitonin serum levels also are prognostically significant and superior to staging according to the TNM and EORTC classifications. For instance, patients with calcitonin doubling times of less than 6 months had 5- and 10-year survival rates of 25% and 8%, as opposed to 92% and 37%, respectively, when these doubling times were 6–24 months. All patients whose calcitonin doubling times were greater than 2 years were alive at a mean follow-up of 9.6 years. Likewise, increased CEA serum levels correlate with tumor stage and prognosis.

Early Diagnosis Through Calcitonin Stimulation

The release of calcitonin triggered by an intravenous bolus injection of pentagastrin, the most widely used provocative agent, sometimes can be unpleasant and cause transient flushing, nausea, tingling in limbs, and chest tightness. Notwithstanding the potential for such adverse events, provocative testing is needed to enable detection of occult medullary thyroid carcinoma.

From a clinical perspective, the main indications for calcitonin stimulation are the following:

1. *Early detection of occult medullary microcarcinomas in patients with nodular goiter which otherwise would go undetected.*

This concept has been instrumental in improving overall survival in patients with sporadic medullary thyroid carcinoma.

2. *Individualized timing of curative pre-emptive thyroidectomy in RET gene carriers.*

In some instances, progression of hereditary medullary thyroid carcinoma can be unexpectedly fast, necessitating thyroidectomy earlier than usually recommended on the basis of RET gene analysis. Determination of basal and pentagastrin-stimulated serum calcitonin levels in asymptomatic RET carriers allows one to capture the transition phase from C cell hyperplasia to medullary thyroid carcinoma, which is marked by increased stimulated, but still normal basal calcitonin levels, and to schedule the patient for early prophylactic thyroidectomy. As long as the basal calcitonin levels remain within normal limits, additional systematic dissection of the central lymph node compartment (Fig. 4.2) may not be required, sparing the patient the excess risk of postoperative hypoparathyroidism attendant to the procedure.

3. *Estimation of postoperative extent and progression of minimal residual disease.*

Serial measurements of pentagastrin-induced stimulation of serum calcitonin can help estimate postoperative extent and progression of minimal residual disease in patients with borderline or mildly elevated basal calcitonin levels. In patients with excessive basal calcitonin levels, calcitonin stimulation may not be needed.

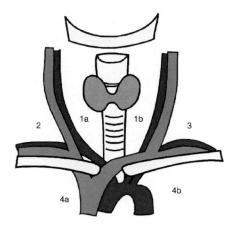

FIGURE 4.2. Dralle's classification of cervicomediastinal lymph node compartments. C1: Central cervical compartment: a, right; b, left. C2: Lateral cervical compartment (right). C3: Lateral cervical compartment (left). C4: Mediastinal compartment (infrabrachiocephalic): a, right; b, left.

DNA-Based RET Analysis – The Diagnostic Gold Standard

The discovery of the RET protooncogene as the susceptibility gene for hereditary medullary thyroid carcinoma and the MEN 2 syndrome was hailed as a great leap forward in the clinical management of RET carriers, quickly elevating DNA-based RET analysis to the rank of a new gold standard. This universal acceptance was enhanced by the identification of genotype-phenotype relationships which continue to transform the clinical management of RET carriers.

1. Barring sample mix up, DNA-based RET analysis is able to correctly identify 95% of RET carriers, sparing unaffected kindreds the stigma and emotional distress associated with heritable disease. Non-carriers can be released from subsequent surveillance, whereas RET carriers can undergo timely thyroidectomy.

2. The well-established genotype-phenotype correlations can be harnessed to individualize the clinical management of RET carriers according to the risk (very high, high, and least high) inherent in the respective RET mutation (Fig. 4.3). The combination of genetic and biochemical information is useful in individualizing surgical intervention in terms of timing and extent of the operation. Limiting the extent of resection decreases potential surgical risks, such as the excess risk of postoperative hypoparathyroidism associated with central lymph node dissection.

3. Genotype-phenotype relationships clarify the risk of the average RET carrier to develop not only medullary thyroid carcinomas, but also pheochromocytomas and primary hyperparathyroidism. Intra- and interfamilial variability can confound the precision of individual predictions based on genetic information. With decreasing RET risk category, the chance of developing additional neuroendocrine tumors diminishes.

Molecular testing is warranted in all patients with seemingly sporadic medullary thyroid carcinomas or adrenal pheochromocytomas. In patients with multiglandular parathyroid disease, a DNA-based test for MEN1 germline mutations may be more appropriate because of the higher prevalence of primary hyperparathyroidism in this condition.

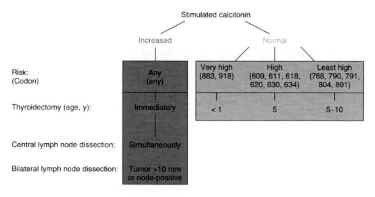

FIGURE 4.3. University of Halle algorithm: timing of thyroidectomy in RET gene carriers.

Tumor Stage – A Most Powerful Indicator of Survival

The largest multivariate analysis of survival undertaken to date encompassed 899 patients with sporadic and hereditary medullary thyroid carcinomas. Altogether, 3- and 5-year survival rates for patients with medullary thyroid carcinoma were 86% and 78%, respectively. 10-year survival was 98% with and 70% without postoperative normalization of serum calcitonin. TNM tumor stage at the time of operation was the most powerful indicator of survival. Normalization of calcitonin levels was solely dependent on tumor stage at the time of surgery.

Tumor stage and extent of disease obviously are reflected by the number of lymph node metastases. Irrespective of location, involvement of 10 and more lymph nodes or of more than two cervicomediastinal lymph node compartments seems to almost always preclude postoperative normalization of serum calcitonin. The rate of postoperative calcitonin normalization may not exceed 60% in patients with node-negative, and 10% in patients with node-positive, tumors.

From these data, the following conclusions can be drawn:

1. Early diagnosis of medullary thyroid carcinomas, as long as they are still confined to the neck, is the only chance to improve outcome. Routine calcitonin screening in patients with nodular goiter is pivotal in advancing the diagnosis of occult medullary thyroid carcinomas.
2. Meticulous compartment-oriented dissection of cervical lymph nodes may increase the rates of postoperative calcitonin normalization more than selective removal of gross lymph node metastases only ("berry picking"). The clinical utility of systematic lymph node dissection is limited when more than 10 lymph nodes or more than two lymph node compartments are involved, conditions which signify systemic disease.

Concept of Locoregional
Spread and Distant Metastases

Dissemination of lymphatic tumor cells through the lymphatic system which drains the thyroid gland is believed to evolve in a stepwise fashion (Fig. 4.4): Lymph node metastasis starts in the central (UICC groups 1, 2, and 8) and the lateral cervical (UICC groups 3 through 7) lymph node compartments on the side of the primary thyroid malignancy. From these regional lymph node groups, lymph node metastases progress to the opposite lateral cervical and the mediastinal lymph node compartment. These latter groups of lymph nodes have been designated as nonregional and "distant" lymph nodes because their involvement is indicative of distant metastasis. This pattern of spread of lymph node metastasis often is blunted on reoperation, where the rate of lymph node metastases is much higher in all cervicomediastinal compartments than in the primary setting.

The ipsilateral cervical lymph node compartments constitute the watershed between local and systemic disease. With strictly ipsilateral lymphatic drainage of tumor cells, surgical

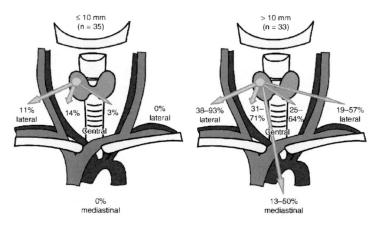

FIGURE 4.4. Pattern of lymph node metastasis by primary size of medullary thyroid carcinoma at initial operation (Data from Machens et al., 2002).

cure can be accomplished through systematic lymph node dissection in some, but not all patients. In stark contrast, extension of lymph node metastasis beyond these ipsilateral lymph nodes into the contralateral neck usually is not curable by the addition of lymph node dissection in the contralateral neck.

Surgical Intervention

Surgery for medullary thyroid carcinoma has never been rigorously evaluated in clinical trials. Major obstacles for conducting prospective studies include:

(a) The relative infrequency of the condition
(b) The comparative longevity of patients in the face of systemic disease
(c) The dilemma of classifying minimal residual disease on the basis of imagining into local and systemic disease

To overcome these obstacles, prohibitively large numbers of patients would need to be enrolled and observed over a prohibitively long period of time.

Considering the wealth of retrospective studies on the subject, the following surgical strategy seems appropriate:

1. The entire thyroid gland should be removed, not only in hereditary, but also in sporadic medullary thyroid carcinoma. Although merely 10% of non-hereditary tumors are multifocal, the sporadic nature of the malignancy often is not recognized until after the operation with the receipt of the genetic test results. When patients with suspected or confirmed medullary thyroid carcinoma are shown preoperatively to have a negative RET gene test, a few surgeons embark on lobectomy instead of thyroidectomy. It is noteworthy that this strategy relies on immunohistological exclusion of tumor multifocality which generally is not available before or during the operation.

2. Because of the high prevalence of central and lateral cervical lymph node metastases on the side of the primary thyroid tumor (already 14% in medullary thyroid

microcarcinoma at the initial operation; Fig. 4.4), these lymph nodes should also be cleared at the initial operation.

3. Although compartment-oriented, systemic lymph node dissection in all likelihood is more effective than selective lymph node dissection ("berry picking"), the expected clinical superiority of this approach has never been formally verified. The main argument supporting systemic lymph node dissection has been the perceived reduction of surgical morbidity because fewer reoperations are then required for residual lymph node metastases.

4. Even though less common, involvement of the opposite lateral cervical and the mediastinal lymph node compartment heralds systemic disease. Although no study so far has compared 3-compartmentectomy with 2-compartmentectomy, most surgical centers prefer 3-compartmentectomy, certainly for tumors larger than 10 mm (Fig. 4.4), with a view of decreasing the number of cervical reoperations for suspected or confirmed residual disease.

5. Transsternal mediastinal lymph node dissection may be needed to alleviate symptoms arising from local compression, or to preempt invasion of adjoining vital structures, such as the mediastinal trachea. As most patients with infrabrachiocephalic tumor extension harbor systemic disease, these mediastinal dissections almost never are curative and therefore are not indicated on a prophylactic basis.

6. In the event of persistent or recurrent disease, the indication for, and the extent of, reoperation is not always straightforward. As a matter of principle, any reoperation should take a compartment-oriented approach. Imaging is essential in pinpointing residual disease to a cervical or mediastinal area. In addition to percutaneous ultrasonography, computerized tomography (CT), magnetic resonance imaging (MRI), and fluoro-deoxyglucose or DOPA positron emission tomography-computerized tomography (FDG-PET-CT or DOPA-PET-CT) can be crucial in delineating recurrent tumor. For diagnosis of laryngeal, tracheal, and esophageal involvement, three-dimensional MRI reconstruction, coupled with endoscopic examinations (tracheoscopy, esophagoscopy), may facilitate planning of the reoperation.

7. For patients with increased calcitonin levels, but without
   demonstrable tumor, a "wait and see" policy maybe appropriate. In this scenario, reoperations should be restricted to
   patients who had inadequate initial operations without systematic lymph node dissection. Although occult metastases
   in this setting are frequently present in the neck, the benefit
   of such reoperations for long-term survival is unclear.

Treatment Options for Systemic Disease

Management of systemic disease which is not amenable to
surgical intervention is first and foremost directed at the
relief of symptoms. Pain control and treatment of diarrhea
can be accomplished with the administration of analgesics
and loperamide. Painful bone metastases to the spine, the
pelvis or the limbs that do not require operative removal or
stabilization may benefit from external radiation to the
respective site.

Often diffuse and multiple, pulmonary, hepatic, and bone
metastases from medullary thyroid carcinoma may occur
alone or in conjunction with one another. In the latter event,
there is a dire need for systemic therapy. Neither radioiodine
treatment nor systemic chemotherapy are particularly effective. Somatostatin analogs and other available modalities pro
duce only rare tumor responses and barely control symptoms.
Gastrin analogs and tyrosine kinase inhibitors hold promise
for targeted therapy of medullary thyroid carcinoma, but have
not yet entered pivotal clinical trials for that indication.
Another promising therapeutic modality is pretargeted radioimmunotherapy based on a bispecific monoclonal anti-CEA
antibody and a iodine-131 bivalent hapten. In a retrospective
study, overall survival was significantly improved (110 vs. 61
months; $P < 0.03$) in high-risk patients who had calcitonin doubling times of less than 2 years. Toxicity was mainly hemato-
logic and related to bone/bone marrow spread.

Selective arterial chemoembolization has been advocated
for the treatment of multiple liver metastases which are irre-
sectable. Partial radiologic tumor responses were achieved in

roughly half of the patients (42–55%) and were associated with liver involvement in less than 30%. Symptomatic response varied from 40–73%, but was usually transient and often lost after more than 12 months since arterial chemoembolization. Before chemoembolization can be contemplated for use in RET carriers or patients with unknown RET carrier status, biochemical and radiological exclusion of concomitant pheochromocytomas is a prerequisite. At least one fatal hypertensive crisis has occurred in a patient with metastatic medullary thyroid carcinoma following the inadvertent chemoembolization of liver metastases from a recurrent pheochromocytoma, the malignancy of which had not been recognized at first adrenalectomy at another institution.

Selected Readings

Barbet J, Campion L, Kraeber-Bodéré F, Chatal JF; GTC Study Group et al. (2005) Prognostic impact of serum calcitonin and carcinoembryonic antigen doubling-times in patients with medullary thyroid carcinoma. J Clin Endocrinol Metab 90:6077–6084

Brandi ML, Gagel RF, Angeli A, et al. (2001) Guidelines for diagnosis and therapy of MEN type 1 and type 2. J Clin Endocrinol Metab 86:5658–5671

Chatal JF, Campion L, Kraeber-Bodéré F, et al. (2006) Survival improvement in patients with medullary thyroid carcinoma who undergo pretargeted anti-carcinoembryonic-antigen radioimmunotherapy: a collaborative study with the French Endocrine Tumor Group. J Clin Oncol 24:1705–1711

Dralle H, Gimm O, Simon D, et al. (1998) Prophylactic thyroidectomy in 75 children and adolescents with hereditary medullary thyroid carcinoma: German and Austrian experience. World J Surg 22:744–751

Dralle H (2002) Lymph node dissection and medullary thyroid carcinoma. Br J Surg 89:1073–1075

Elisei R, Bottici V, Luchetti F, et al. (2004) Impact of routine measurement of serum calcitonin on the diagnosis and outcome of medullary thyroid cancer: experience in 10.864 patients with nodular thyroid disorders. J Clin Endocrinol Metab 89:163–168

Fleming JB, Lee JE, Bouvet M, et al. (1999) Surgical strategy for the treatment of medullary thyroid carcinoma. Ann Surg 230:697–707

Fromigué J, Baere D, Baudin E, et al. (2006) Chemoembolization for liver metastases from medullary thyroid carcinoma. J Clin Endocrinol Metab 91:2496–2499

Karges W, Dralle H, Raue F, et al. (2004) Calcitonin measurement to detect medullary thyroid carcinoma in nodular goiter: German evidence-based consensus recommendation. Exp Clin Endocrinol Diabet 112:52–58

Machens A, Gimm O, Ukkat J, et al. (2000) Improved prediction of calcitonin normalization in medullary thyroid carcinoma patients by quantitative lymph node analysis. Cancer 88:1909–1915

Machens A, Hinze R, Thomusch O, Dralle H (2002) Pattern of nodal metastasis for primary and reoperative thyroid cancer. World J Surg 26:22–28

Machens A, Niccoli-Sire P, Hoegel J, et al. (2003) Early malignant progression of hereditary medullary thyroid cancer. N Engl J Med 349:1517–1525

Machens A, Schneyer U, Holzhausen HJ, Dralle H (2005) Prospects of remission in medullary thyroid carcinoma according to basal calcitonin level. J Clin Endocrinol Metab 90:2029–2034

Machens A, Ukkat J, Brauckhoff M, et al. (2005) Advances in the management of hereditary medullary thyroid cancer. J Intern Med 257:50–59

Machens A, Brauckhoff M, Holzhausen HJ, et al. (2005) Codon-specific development of pheochromocytoma in multiple endocrine neoplasia type 2. J Clin Endocrinol Metab 90:3999–4003

Machens A, Holzhausen HJ, Dralle H (2006) Contralateral cervical and mediastinal lymph node metastasis in medullary thyroid cancer: systemic disease? Surgery 139:28–32

Modigliani E, Cohen R, Compos JM, et al. (1998) Prognostic factors for survival and for biochemical cure in medullary thyroid carcinoma: results in 899 patients. Clin Endocrinol 48:265–273

Moley JF, DeBenedetti MK (1999) Patterns of nodal metastases in palpable medullary thyroid carcinoma. Recommendations for extent of node dissection. Ann Surg 229:880–887; discussion 887–888

5
Hyperparathyroidism: Primary and Secondary

Herbert Chen

Pearls and Pitfalls

- Operative treatment (parathyroidectomy) is considered the principal therapy for all patients with primary hyperparathyroidism (HPT).
- Eighty percent of patients with primary HPT have parathyroid adenomas and thus are candidates for minimally invasive parathyroidectomy (MIP).
- Preoperative localization is essential for MIP and reoperative cases. Sestamibi scanning is the best technique.
- MIP is not appropriate for patients with HPT due to multiple endocrine neoplasia (MEN) type I. The preferred operation is total parathyroidectomy, parathyroid autotransplantation to the nondominant forearm, bilateral cervical thymectomy, and cryopreservation.
- The most commonly missed location for a parathyroid gland is the retroesophageal area. Other ectopic areas include the thymus, carotid sheaths, and intrathyroidal.
- Intraoperative parathyroid hormone (PTH) testing can predict cure in patients with primary and tertiary HPT. A drop of >50% after 5 or 10 min indicates adequate resection.
- Parathyroid cancer should be considered in patients with primary HPT, a serum calcium >14.0 mg/dl, and a hard, palpable neck mass.

K.I. Bland et al. (eds.), *Endocrine Surgery*,
DOI: 10.1007/978-1-84996-447-0_5,
© Springer-Verlag London Limited 2011

- Mediastinal parathyroid adenomas occur 2–5% of the time. Most can be resected from the neck with a cervical thymectomy. VATS surgery (with radioguidance) is the optimal treatment for mediastinal parathyroid adenomas below the aortic arch.
- Calciphylaxis is an urgent indication for total parathyroidectomy in patients with secondary HPT.
- In patients with tertiary HPT after renal transplantation, subtotal parathyroidectomy is the operation of choice.
- Cryopreservation should be performed in cases of reoperative parathyroid surgery and in patients with parathyroid hyperplasia.

Sir Richard Owen first identified the parathyroid gland during an autopsy of an Indian rhinoceros at the London Zoo in 1850. Ivar Sandstrom, a Swedish medical student, later reported the first gross and histologic description of the glands in humans. A normal human parathyroid gland weighs between 30 and 50 mg, and almost all patients have at least four parathyroid glands: two upper parathyroids derived from the IV branchial pouch and two lower parathyroids derived from the III branchial pouch. The blood supply of the parathyroid glands is usually from the inferior thyroid artery.

Primary Hyperparathyroidism

Presentation. Primary HPT has an incidence of 0.1–0.5% in the general population, affects up to 2% of the elderly, and is most common in postmenopausal women. Historically, patients with this disease presented with symptoms of bone disease or kidney stones. Since the development of serum chemistry auto-analyzers, hypercalcemia identified on routine laboratory testing has become the most common presentation of primary HPT. However, the vast majority of patients with HPT will have subjective, identifiable symptoms, which are varied and are often difficult to appreciate due to their lack of specificity. These include cardiovascular (hypertension), gastrointestinal (nausea, vomiting, anorexia, constipation, abdominal pain, pancreatitis), renal (nephrocalcinosis, nephrolithiasis, calciuria, polyuria, overflow incontinence), psychiatric (depression, anxiety, psychosis), skeletal (osteitis fibrosa cystica, osteopenia/osteoporosis, bone pain, pathological fractures), and neuromuscular (fatigue, myalgias, muscle weakness) signs or symptoms. Patients may present with an acute hypercalcemic crisis (calcium >14.0 mg/dl). The symptoms of hypercalcemic crisis include the rapid onset of nausea, vomiting, weight loss, fatigue, weakness, and confusion.

Diagnosis. The laboratory diagnosis of primary HPT consists of an elevated serum calcium level in conjunction with an inappropriately high normal or elevated PTH level. Other associated laboratory abnormalities include: hypophosphatemia (50%), hypomagnesemia (5–10%), and an elevated alkaline phosphatase, a marker for bone disease. Many patients will have a chloride-to-phosphate ratio greater than 30. Urinary calcium levels are either normal or elevated. In patients with a low urinary calcium level(<50 mg/24 h), familial hypocalciuric hypercalcemia should be ruled out. Bone mineral densitometry can help determine the effects of HPT on bone loss and assess the need for operative intervention. Primary HPT is caused by a single adenoma in approximately 80% of patients, double adenomas in 5–10%, and hyperplasia in 10–15%. Less than 1% of patients will have parathyroid carcinoma. PrimaryHPT can be part of several genetic syndromes, most notably the MEN syndromes. Nearly 100% of patients with MEN I will develop primary HPT, which is due to parathyroid hyperplasia. Primary HPT is less frequently seen in MEN IIa, occurring in approximately 25% of cases.

Operative indications. Surgery is the only curative treatment for primary HPT. In experienced hands the cure rate of parathyroidectomy is >95% with a long-term complication rate of <5% (permanent hypoparathyroidism<2%, permanent recurrent laryngeal nerve [RLN] injury <2%).We believe that all patients with primary HPT should be referred to an experienced surgeon for consideration of parathyroidectomy.

Our preference is to offer surgical intervention to all patients who do not have prohibitive medical comorbidities. Studies have shown a significant increase in bone mineral densities, an improvement in subtle neurocognitive symptoms, a reduction in fatigue, a decrease in premature cardiovascular death, and an improved quality of life in patients with primary HPT after parathyroidectomy. Despite the potential benefits of surgery, others prefer a more conservative approach. A summary of indications for surgery in patients with primary HPT is summarized in Table 5.1. Clearly, any symptomatic patient should be considered for surgical intervention. Patients who do not present with classical symptoms are frequently labeled as asymptomatic. The NIH consensus guidelines for the management of these asymptomatic patients with primary HPT were revised in 2002, and are included in Table 5.1. These indications include young age, moderate to severe hypercalcemia, hypercalcuria, and osteopenia. In addition, many asymptomatic patients may prefer surgical invention as opposed to observation.

Preoperative considerations. Most patients with primary HPT have modest hypercalcemia and do not need any

TABLE 5.1. Indications for surgery in patients with primary HPT.

1. Symptoms or signs of disease (hypertension, nausea, vomiting, anorexia, constipation, abdominal pain, pancreatitis, nephrocalcinosis, nephrolithiasis, calciuria, polyuria, overflow incontinence, depression, anxiety, psychosis, osteitis fibrosa cystica, osteopenia/osteoporosis, bone pain, pathological fractures, fatigue, myalgias, muscle weakness)

2. Serum calcium greater or equal to 1 mg/dl above the normal range

3. Urine calcium excretion > 400 mg/24 h

4. Reduction in bone mass marked by a t-score < –2.0 at any site (lumbar spine, hip, or forearm)

5. Age 50 years or less

6. Reduction in creatinine clearance by >30%

7. Medical surveillance is neither desirable nor possible

8. Patient preference

preoperative medical intervention. However, patients with severe hypercalcemia (crisis) require urgent medical treatment prior to surgery. The first goal in the treatment of hypercalcemic crisis is to increase the excretion of calcium. This is done first by rehydrating the patient intravenously with normal saline, followed by diuresis with a loop diuretic (Lasix). The second goal of treatment is to inhibit bone resorption with bisphosphonates. Bisphosphonates inhibit osteoclast function and start working within 3–6 days with their effects lasting weeks. In most cases prompt parathyroidectomy after hydration is preferred over bisphosphonates due to the prolonged postoperative hypocalcemia that can occur after the use of these drugs. Calcimimetic agents, such as cinacalcet, are now available clinically for the treatment of intractable HPT. These drugs reduce circulating PTH levels by increasing the sensitivity of the CaR to extracellular calcium. The indications for the use of this new class of drugs are still evolving.

Parathyroid Localization

Preoperative Imaging

Sestamibi scans. Parathyroid localization is essential for patients undergoing minimally invasive parathyroid surgical approaches (see the following), as well as patients having reoperative neck exploration. Our preferred imaging approach for patients having initial parathyroid surgery is shown in the treatment algorithm(Fig. 5.1). The most commonly performed and the first-line imaging test at our institution is a Tc-99m sestamibi scan. Tc-99m sestamibi scans can be performed with planar and oblique images, with single photon emission computed tomography(SPECT), or with CT fusion (Fig. 5.2). The advantages of Tc-99m sestamibi are its high sensitivity (70–80%), availability, 3-D anatomic reconstruction capacity, and the ability to evaluate ectopic locations such as the mediastinum concurrently.

Subtraction scans. In patients who prefer a minimally invasive procedure but have negative sestamibi scans, we consider

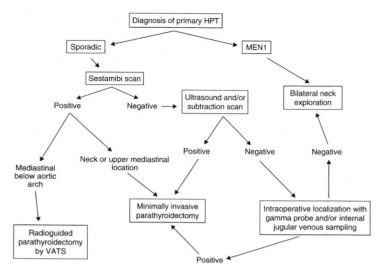

FIGURE 5.1. Imaging and treatment algorithm for patients with primary HPT.

additional imaging, including thallium pertechnetate/Tc-99m sestamibi subtraction scanning. Thallium pertechnetate/Tc-99m sestamibi subtraction scanning is an alternative nuclear imaging modality that has been used with some success with a sensitivity around 75%.

Ultrasound. Ultrasound is another commonly used imaging modality. It is noninvasive and inexpensive, but very operator-dependent. Ultrasound is frequently used as an adjunct to confirm a finding on another imaging modality. When combined with Tc-99m sestamibi, the combined sensitivity is >90%. In addition, lesions that are suspicious for hyperplastic parathyroid tissue can be confirmed with fine needle aspiration under ultrasound guidance.

Other. In reoperative patients, we consider other imaging tests including CT and MRI. These tests are more expensive and less sensitive at localizing a parathyroid within the anterior neck, but can be useful in identifying abnormalities deep within the neck or mediastinum. More invasive localization tools, such as arteriography and venography, are often useful for patients with recurrent or persistent HPT and negative noninvasive studies.

Intraoperative Localization

Intraoperative ultrasound. In addition to preoperative imaging studies, there are several intraoperative adjuncts which are useful to aid in the localization of abnormal parathyroid glands, particularly in the patient with negative imaging. Many surgeons utilize intraoperative ultrasound to evaluate

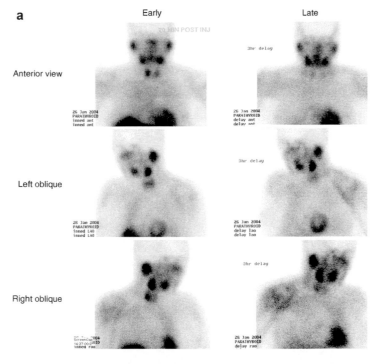

FIGURE 5.2. Tc-99m sestamibi scans indicating a single parathyroid adenoma. (**a**) Planar images (right upper adenoma); (**b**) SPECT images (left lower adenoma); (**c**) with fused CT images (right lower adenoma).

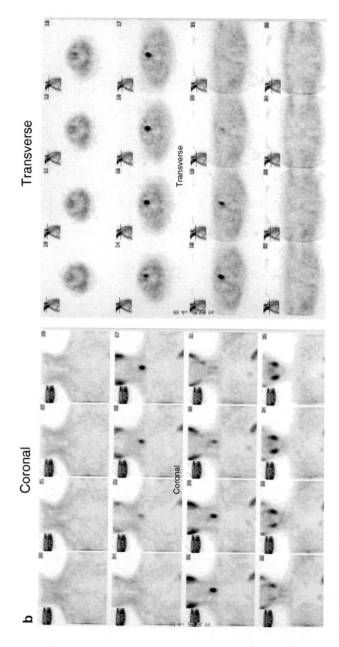

FIGURE 5.2. (continued).

Anterior   Lateral   Transverse

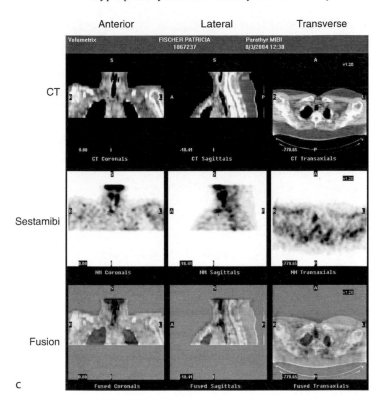

C

FIGURE 5.2. (continued).

the neck during thyroid and parathyroid surgery. This can provide useful anatomic information.

Radioguided parathyroidectomy. Intraoperative gamma probe localization relies on the fact that there is variable sestamibi uptake in the thyroid compared to abnormal parathyroid tissue. Patients typically receive a preoperative injection of 10 mCi of Tc-99m sestamibi 1–2 h prior to being taken to surgery. A 11-mm gamma probe is used intraoperatively to guide incision placement as well as to direct the dissection, allowing the surgeon to focus in on the location of the abnormal parathyroid tissue. The gamma probe is then used to confirm that the tissue resected is indeed parathyroid tissue.

Counts >20% of background are considered diagnostic for parathyroid tissue. The benefits of the intraoperative gamma probe have been controversial. In our experience, the gamma probe has been useful in the majority of patients by reducing operative time and minimizing the extent of dissection. Furthermore, the technology can be used for patients with primary, secondary, or tertiary HPT.

Bilateral internal jugular venous sampling and PTH testing. Another emerging technique is internal jugular venous sampling with rapid PTH testing. In patients with negative imaging studies and difficult-to-find parathyroid glands, blood from both internal jugular veins can be sampled and tested for PTH levels utilizing intraoperative PTH testing (see next section).A gradient of >5% between the two internal veins suggests the presence of a parathyroid adenoma on the higher side with a positive predictive value of 70%.

Primary HPT: Operative Approaches

Open Bilateral Neck Exploration

Background. The standard surgical approach to HPT has been a bilateral neck exploration. This technique is highly successful with cure rates of 95% in experienced hands. The long-term complication rate of a bilateral neck exploration is low(<5%), but the incidence of transient hypocalcemia can be as high as 30%. This technique is dependent upon the successful identification of all four parathyroid glands and requires surgeon expertise in the recognition of the parathyroid glands in their normal and ectopic locations. No preoperative localization is necessary.Although special intraoperative adjuncts are not required, we find the gamma probe and intraoperative PTH testing very helpful during bilateral neck explorations (see minimally invasive parathyroidectomy section).

Technique. At our institution, the patient is positioned on the operating room table in a beach chair position with their arms tucked. An inflatable pressure bag is placed under the shoulders to expose the neck. A 2–4-cm incision is made one fingerbreadth below the cricoid cartilage. The strap muscles are divided down their midline and the thyroid is exposed. The variations seen in the locations of the parathyroid glands are based mostly on their embryogenesis. The inferior glands descend with the thymus and can be found anywhere from the larynx to the mediastinum. Inferior glands are most frequently located just posterior to the inferior lobe of the thyroid gland and anterior and medial to the RLN. They can be displaced inferiorly and located within the thymus or anterior mediastinum, or located more posterior within the tracheoesophageal groove. Eighty percent of all inferior glands are located within 2 cm of the inferior pole of the thyroid. The superior glands are typically located posterior to the upper pole of the thyroid near the point the RLN enters the larynx. The gland is most commonly located posterior and lateral to the RLN. Because the incidence of multiple gland disease is as high as 20%, it is essential to make every effort to identify all four parathyroid glands. In the presence of one, two, or three enlarged adenomatous glands, these abnormal glands should be resected and the normal appearing gland(s) left in situ. If all four glands are enlarged, then the treatment options are a subtotal (3 1/2 gland) parathyroidectomy or a total parathyroidectomy with autotransplantation to the nondominant forearm.

Minimally Invasive Parathyroidectomy

Background. Since the majority of patients with primary HPT have only a single adenoma (80–85%), attempts have been made to minimize the extent of surgery. MIP consists of identifying and resecting a single abnormal gland without visualizing the remaining normal parathyroid glands. The central component of this technique is accurate preoperative localization. A second component is radioguided gamma probe detection. The last, and perhaps most important component, is intraoperative PTH testing. The use of intraoperative PTH testing allows determination of biochemical cure at the time of surgery. This is based upon the principle that PTH has a half-life of 2–4 min. Hence, within 5–10 min of resecting a single adenoma, over half of the PTH in the bloodstream will have been cleared, since the other three normal glands will be suppressed. However, if another hyperfunctioning parathyroid gland is present, the PTH levels will not fall by 50%. Therefore, intraoperative PTH testing can replace intraoperative visualization of the other parathyroid glands by effectively measuring residual PTH secretion from the remaining glands. Intraoperative PTH testing has been shown to improve the cure rate of MIP and expands the population of patients who are candidates for MIP.

Technique. In order to consider for a MIP, a patient must have undergone preoperative imaging that reveals a single abnormal gland. One to two hours prior to surgery, the patient is given an IV injection of 10 mCi of Tc-99m sestamibi, which is used intraoperatively to help localize the parathyroid tissue. The patient is positioned the same as with conventional exploration. An additional large bore peripheral IV is placed for blood draws for intraoperative PTH testing. If local anesthesia is, a superficial cervical block is performed at this time with 1% lidocaine. Sedation with either midazolam or propofol may be used to aid in patient comfort. Prior to making an incision, a baseline PTH level is drawn from the patient's peripheral IV line. An 11-mm collimated gamma probe (Neoprobe 2000, Ethicon Endo-Surgery, Cincinnati, Ohio) is then utilized. Since both the thyroid and the parathyroid take up Tc-99m sestamibi, the background count is set over the thyroid isthmus. Our standard incision is 2 cm in length and is placed in the midline transversely. The strap muscles are divided down the middle and the thyroid is exposed. The gamma probe is then used to focus our dissection to the area of highest uptake. The abnormal parathyroid is identified and its vascular pedicle clipped. The adenoma is then resected and ex vivo counts of the tissue are obtained by placing the gland atop the gamma probe. Ex vivo counts >20% of background are consistent with parathyroid tissue.

After confirming that parathyroid tissue was removed, the intraoperative PTH assay is then used to determine the adequacy of the resection. Intraoperative PTH levels are obtained 5, 10, and 15 min after resection of the abnormal gland. Our criteria is a 50% drop from our baseline PTH level as the definition of an adequate resection. If there is not a 50% drop in PTH levels at 5, 10, or 15 min, then the ipsilateral parathyroid gland is visualized and, if abnormal, resected. Intraoperative PTH levels are again used to confirm that there is no additional disease. If the ipsilateral gland is normal or the PTH does not fall after resection of the second gland, a bilateral exploration is performed. All four parathyroid glands are identified and any abnormal parathyroid tissue is resected.

Benefits. There have been several reports showing that the cure rate of MIP appears to be equal, if not better, than bilateral neck exploration. There are several advantages of MIP. The incidence of symptomatic postoperative hypocalcemia has been shown to be reduced from 25% in a bilateral exploration to 7% with MIP. The ability to perform a MIP under local anesthesia is especially important in the elderly population, who are at higher risk for general anesthetic complications. In addition, using local anesthesia allows assessment of RLN function by having the patient talk during the surgical procedure. A smaller incision size leads to improved cosmesis and potentially less postoperative pain. MIP has been shown to reduce operating room time by up to 50%. Most patients can safely be discharged on the same day, leading to a reduction in hospital length of stay and a potential overall cost savings.

Mediastinal Parathyroid Adenomas

Background. Mediastinal parathyroid adenomas occur in approximately 2–5% of patients with primary HPT. The vast majority of these lesions are present within the thymus gland and can be resected via a cervical approach with or without cervical thymectomy. However, those below the level of the aortic arch are difficult to access through the neck. In the past, these patients have required a median sternotomy for resection. However, in the absence of previous lung surgery, most patients with these mid to low mediastinal parathyroid adenomas can be treated with a minimally invasive thoracic approach: VATS resection.

Radioguided parathyroidectomy via VATS technique. Ten mCi of Tc-99m sestamibi is administered 1–2 h preoperatively. After induction of anesthesia, single lung ventilation is achieved using a double lumen endotracheal tube. Two 5-mm ports are placed in the fourth and seventh intercostal spaces in the posterior axillary line and one 11.5-mm port in the fourth intercostal space in the midclavicular line; the latter is used to introduce a sterile gamma probe. The background counts are measured on the distal lung while compressed. During VATS, the lung is used rather than the thyroid, and provides the background counts reflecting uptake in normal tissues. The mediastinal tissues are then scanned with the gamma probe looking for counts above the background counts to determine the exact location of the parathyroid adenoma in the chest. After localization with the gamma probe, the adenoma is resected with a harmonic scalpel. Excision of parathyroid tissue is confirmed by an ex vivo count >20% of the background counts. Blood is then sampled at 5, 10, and 15 min after resection for PTH. If a >50% drop in PTH levels occurs, then the operation is terminated. If the PTH level fails to fall, the surgeon then explores the neck for a second adenoma or additional hyperplasic glands. Following resection of the second adenoma and/or other enlarged parathyroids, the PTH level is checked again after an additional 5 and 10 min. A 24F chest tube is placed prior to closure.

Other Considerations

Multiple endocrine neoplasia type I (MEN I). Patients with MEN I virtually all have four-gland hyperplasia. In these patients, we do not routinely obtain preoperative imaging scans, but utilize bilateral neck exploration with radioguided techniques. We identify and resect all four parathyroid glands and perform bilateral cervical thymectomies. The latter procedure resects potential supernumerary parathyroid glands, as well as thymic carcinoids, which can be present in these patients. We then transplant 10–12 1 × 3 mm parathyroid fragments into the nondominant brachioradialis muscle. The remaining parathyroid tissue is cryopreserved. Because patients will be hypocalcemic postoperatively until their forearm grafts begin to function, they are immediately started on calcium and calcitriol.

Parathyroid cancer. Less than 1% of patients with primary HPT will have parathyroid cancer. This should be suspected in patients who present with a palpable, hard mass and a serum calcium >14 mg/dl. Operative treatment should consist of an en bloc resection and ipsilateral thyroid lobectomy. If clinically enlarged lymph nodes are present, an ipsilateral central node dissection should be performed.

The "missing" parathyroid gland. Occasionally, hyperfunctioning parathyroidgland(s) cannot be identified at the time of neck exploration. In these cases, it is important to identify and not injure the normal parathyroid glands, and to determine which of the four parathyroid glands is "missing." In these cases, testing blood with intraoperative PTH levels from different locations of both internal jugular veins can often provide localizing information. If an inferior parathyroid gland is missing, then an ipsilateral cervical thymectomy should be performed because up to 15% of lower glands are located within the thymus or between the thyroid and thymus. Then, the carotid sheath on that side should be opened to the level of the bifurcation. A final option is to obtain an intraoperative ultrasound of the thyroid looking for an intrathyroidal parathyroid adenoma, which occurs in 1–4% of cases. A blind thyroid lobectomy should not be performed. If a superior gland is missing, then the tracheoesophageal groove and retropharyngeal space should be explored, taking care to avoid injuring the RLN. The goal of the first exploration is to clear the neck of any disease. However, if no abnormal parathyroid tissue is identified after a thorough exploration, it is important for the surgeon to meticulously document which parathyroids were identified and what areas were explored in the search for the missing gland. Normal-appearing parathyroid glands should never be removed. Median sternotomy and mediastinal exploration, in the absence of definitive preoperative localization to the medi-astinum, should never be pursued at the initial exploration. In these cases, the operation should be terminated and the patient reimaged at a later date.

Recurrent or persistent disease. Cure after parathyroidec-tomy is typically defined as normocalcemia at least 6 months postoperatively. Biochemical HPT within 6 months of sur-gery is termed persistent disease. Persistent disease is typi-cally due to failure to identify the causative adenoma, a missed second adenoma, or inadequately resected hyperpla-sia. Recurrent disease is most commonly due to growth of hyperplastic tissue left at the original surgery. The key to minimizing the risks of parathyroid surgery is to avoid reop-erative surgery, by performing an adequate operation at the first exploration. Reoperative surgery carries greater risks and the indications for operative intervention must be clear. Localization studies, while optional for an initial exploration, are mandatory prior to pursuing a reexploration. Generally, two concordant imaging localizing studies should be sought prior to offering any patient a reexploration. If noninvasive studies are nonlocalizing or discordant, then invasive local-ization procedures, such as selective arteriography and venous sampling, are justified prior to pursuing reoperative neck surgery.

Secondary HPT

Etiology. The most common cause of secondary HPT is chronic renal failure. Other causes include malabsorption, osteomalacia, and rickets. In renal failure, parathyroid glands become hyperplastic in response to prolonged hypocalcemia, which is a consequence of diminished synthesis of calcitriol, phosphate retention, and resistance of bone to PTH. Thus, in most patients with renal failure, appropriate calcium supplementation with oral calcitriol and vitamin D therapy can adequately control PTH secretion. However, it is often said that "the best treatment of secondary HPT is kidney transplantation." Most patients with secondary HPT can be medically controlled prior to transplantation. With the advent of calcimimetic agents, such as cinacalcet, even patients refractory to traditional calcium and vitamin D replacement can be successfully bridged to transplantation. However, surgery still plays an important role in the management of many patients with secondary HPT.

Indications for parathyroidectomy. The indications for parathyroidectomy in patients with secondary HPT are listed in Table 5.2. An urgent and absolute indication for parathyroidectomy is calciphylaxis, which occurs in up to 4% of patients with secondary HPT. Calciphylaxis usually presents with intensely painful areas of superficial, violaceous mottling, resembling purpura or livedo reticularis (Fig. 5.3). The superficial lesions often present suddenly and progress

TABLE 5.2. Indications for surgery in patients with secondary HPT.

1. Calciphylaxis

2. Failure of medical management and (one of the following):

   (a) Hypercalcemia

   (b) PTH > 800 pg/ml

   (c) Hypercalcuria

   (d) Pruritis

   (e) Pathologic bone fracture

   (f) Osteoporosis

   (g) Ectopic soft tissue calcifications

   (h) Severe vascular calcifications

   (i) Bone pain

   (j) Hyperphosphatemia

3. Patient preference

4. Medical surveillance is neither desired nor possible

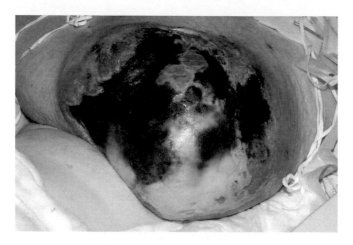

FIGURE 5.3. Skin lesions in a patient with calciphylaxis due to secondary HPT.

rapidly to cutaneous necrosis and dry gangrene. Lesions most commonly develop on the extremities or trunk, but involvement of penis, breast, digits, muscle, and bowel have been reported. Significant mortality, reported as high as 87% in some studies, often results from wound expansion and barrier breakdown, leading to sepsis. Diagnosis is made by elevated PTH and biopsy of the skin lesions. Prompt total parathyroidectomy has been shown to improve survival and accelerate wound healing in these patients. Other indications for parathyroidectomy in patients with secondary HPT are failure of medical management, accompanied by one of the following, including hypercalcemia, hypercalcuria, PTH >800 pg/ml, pruritus, ectopic soft tissue calcifications, and severe vascular calcifications(Table 5.2).

Operative management. Since virtually all patients with secondary HPT will have four-gland hyperplasia, we do not use preoperative parathyroid imaging. Bilateral neck explorations and identification of all four enlarged parathyroid glands are performed. Our preference is four-gland resection (total parathyroidectomy). A 10–12 1 × 3 mm parathyroid fragment is then transplanted into the nondominant brachioradialis muscle. (In patients with calciphylaxis, no parathyroid autotransplantation is performed.) The remaining parathyroid tissue is cryopreserved. Because patients will be hypocalcemic postoperatively until their forearm grafts begin to function, they are immediately started on calcium and calcitriol.

Tertiary HPT

Etiology. Tertiary HPT is the term often used to describe a patient who has hyperfunction of the parathyroid glands that continues or becomes apparent after kidney transplantation. It occurs in approximately 3–5% of patients after renal transplantation. Patients present with elevated calcium and PTH levels after renal transplantation.

Indication for parathyroidectomy. The only reliable cure for tertiary HPT remains surgical excision. The indications for parathyroidectomy in patients with tertiary HPT include: (1) a serum calcium level >12 mg/dl at any time after transplantation, (2) severe osteopenia, (3) symptoms (bone pain, fatigue, pruritus, fractures, mental status changes), (4) a history of renal calculi, or (5) a serum calcium level >10.2 mg/dl more than 1 year after renal transplantation.

Operative management. We recommend bilateral neck exploration in all patients with tertiary HPT. While the majority of patients will have four-gland hyperplasia, about 10% will have only one or two enlarged glands (single or double adenomas). In these patients, we recommend resection of the enlarged glands only. This is based upon our long-term experience with these patients. In patients with four-gland disease, we prefer subtotal parathyroidectomy. In our experience, subtotal parathyroidectomy is associated with a 1% recurrence rate and minimal morbidity. However, total parathyroidectomy with forearm implantation is also an option. We have also shown that intraoperative PTH testing is useful in these patients to accurately predict the extent of resection, with a fall in intraoperative PTH levels of >50% at 10 min predicting cure. Furthermore, we have also shown that radioguided surgery is feasible and potentially beneficial in these patients. Radioguided parathyroidectomy, if available, has been shown to decrease operative time and is helpful in identifying glands in aberrant locations.

Selected Readings

Chen H (2004) Radioguided parathyroid surgery. In: Cameron JL (ed) Advances in surgery. Elsevier, Philadelphia, pp. 377–392

Chen H, Mack E, Starling JR (2005) A comprehensive evaluation of peri-operative adjuncts during minimally invasive parathyroidectomy: which is most reliable? Ann Surg 242:375–383

Chen H, Mack E, Starling JR (2003) Radioguided parathyroidectomy is equally effective for both adenomatous and hyperplastic glands. Ann Surg 238:332–338

Chen H, Pruhs ZM, Starling JR, Mack E (2005) Intraoperative parathyroid hormone testing improves cure rates in patients undergoing minimally invasive parathyroidectomy. Surgery 138:583–590

Chen H, Sokoll L, Udelsman R (1999) Outpatient minimally invasive parathyroidectomy: a combination of sestamibi-SPECT localization, cervical block anesthesia, and intraoperative PTH assay. Surgery 126:14–18

Duffy A, Schurr M, Warner T, Chen H (2006) Long-term outcomes in patients with calciphylaxis from hyperparathyroidism. Annals Surg Oncol 13:96–102

Haustein SV, Mack E, Starling JR, Chen H (2005) The role of intraoperative parathyroid hormone testing in patients with tertiary hyperparathyroidism after renal transplantation. Surgery 138:1066–1071

Nichol PF, Mack E, Bianco J, et al. (2003) Radioguided parathyroidectomy in patients with secondary and tertiary hyperparathyroidism. Surgery 134:713–717

Nichol PF, Starling JR, Mack E, et al. (2002) Long-term follow-up of patients with tertiary hyperparathyroidism treated by resection of a single or double adenoma. Ann Surg 235:673–680

Sippel RS, Bianco JA, Wilson M, et al. (2004) Can thallium-pertechnetate subtraction scanning play a role in the pre-operative imaging for minimally invasive parathyroidectomy? Clin Nucl Med 29:21–26

6
Functioning and Non-functioning Adrenal Tumors

James A. Lee and Quan-Yang Duh

Pearls and Pitfalls

- When faced with an adrenal tumor, the main goals are to determine if it is functional and if it is malignant
- Never biopsy an adrenal tumor until you have ruled out pheochromocytoma
- Fine needle aspiration biopsy is NOT a safe means of diagnosing a pheochromocytoma
- Prior to resection of any adrenal tumor, you must rule out pheochromocytoma and Cushing's syndrome
- When preparing a patient with pheochromocytoma for an operation, you must start with alpha blockade and fluid resuscitation followed by beta blockade as necessary
- Post-operatively, you must stop all potassium supplementation and spironolactone in patients who have had an adrenalectomy for aldosteronoma
- In patients with adrenal Cushing's syndrome, the contralateral adrenal gland is often suppressed and may remain so for weeks to months after the operation. Patients should receive stress dose steroids followed by a taper
- Virilizing or feminizing adrenal neoplasms should be considered to be adrenocortical cancers until proven otherwise
- Complete resection is the only chance for long-term survival in patients with adrenocortical cancer

K.I. Bland et al. (eds.), *Endocrine Surgery*,
DOI: 10.1007/978-1-84996-447-0_6,
© Springer-Verlag London Limited 2011

- Adrenal incidentalomas should be resected if they are functional or larger than5 cm or if they are between 3 to 5 cm in young, healthy patients
- The treatment of non-malignant adrenal neoplasms and solitary metastasis of the adrenal gland is laparoscopic adrenalectomy

Introduction

The adrenal glands are retroperitoneal organs that are divided into the medulla that secretes catecholamines and the cortex that secretes steroid hormones. The cortex makes up 80% of the adrenal volume and is further divided into the zona glomerulosa (which produces aldosterone) and the zona fasciculata and reticularis (which produce glucocorticoids and sex hormones). Neoplasms of the adrenal gland fall into one of six major categories that may overlap in location and hormonal function: aldosteronoma, cortisol-producing neoplasm (Cushing's Syndrome), pheochromocytoma, adrenocortical cancer, metastatic disease, and non-functioning adenoma. Currently, many adrenal neoplasms present as incidentalomas (a clinically inapparent, asymptomatic mass found on imaging done for another reason; see Fig. 6.1 below). Most often, these tumors are readily differentiated based on a thorough history and physical examination, laboratory testing, and computed tomography (CT) scan. The primary goals of evaluation are to determine whether the tumor is functional and whether it is malignant. Functional neoplasms and those with a high malignant potential should be resected.

Pheochromocytoma

Pheochromocytomas are uncommon neoplasms with an annual incidence of 2–8 cases per million and cause hypertension in about 1% of hypertensive patients. Pheochromocytomas are also known as the "10% tumor" because approximately 10% are bilateral, 10% are malignant, 10% are extra-adrenal,

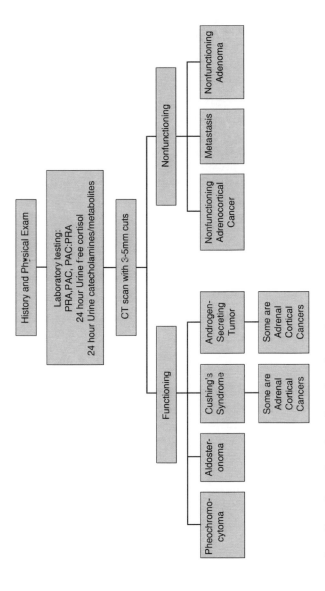

FIGURE 6.1. Overview of work-up for adrenal neoplasms.

10% occur in children, and 10% are familial. Over 90% of pheochromocytomas are sporadic neoplasms without any family history of endocrinopathy. The classic signs and symptoms ascribed to pheochromocytoma include headache, sweating, palpitations, and episodic hypertension. Hypertension can be severe or mild, episodic or chromic. Often symptoms may be precipitated by manipulation of the neoplasm or with other stimuli such as exercise, sexual intercourse, alcohol consumption, or defecation. Occasionally, patients may present in "pheo crisis" in which these symptoms are exaggerated, during which complete cardiac collapse may occur due to myocardial infarction. Such crises and even death have occurred post-partum or during diagnostic biopsy and even minor surgical procedures. It is critically important to avoid invasive procedures and direct manipulation of the mass until the patient has either been ruled out for pheochromocytoma or has been prepared adequately by systemic, pharmacologic alpha blockade.

Screening for pheochromocytoma should be undertaken in the following patient groups: classic symptomatology, unusually labile hypertension, pregnant patients with new-onset hypertension, children with hypertension, adrenal incidentalomas, a family history of pheochromocytoma, and certain genetic syndromes (such as MEN 2A, MEN 2B, and von Hippel-Lindau syndrome). The most common general screening test for pheochromocytoma involves a 24-h urine collection for metanephrines and catecholamines which offers a very acceptable sensitivity of 90% and an excellent specificity of 99%. Measurement of plasma metanephrines is more sensitive (96%) but less specific (85%) and is used generally to screen patients with a high likelihood of having pheochromocytoma (i.e., patients with a personal or family history of pheochromocytoma or a genetic syndrome). Provocative testing has been largely abandoned, because such testing does not increase the diagnostic yield but may precipitate a "pheo crisis." Prior to obtaining a 24-h urine sample, it is important to avoid certain medications or other diagnostic tests that will interfere with accurate testing such as renal failure, iodinated contrast agents (which falsely lower metanephrines levels), and tricyclic anti-depressants, levodopa, and alpha- and beta-blockers. Clear increases in urine metanephrines and catecholamines (greater than two times baseline) are diagnostic of pheochromocytoma. In our series, up to one-third of patients with 1–2 times increase in urine metanephrines and catecholamines have a pheochromocytoma. As such, we recommend alpha blockade or further diagnostic work-up (i.e., metaiodobenzylguanidine (MIBG) scan or plasma metanephrines) for this group of patients. Finally, patients with paragangliomas usually have a high concentrations of urine norepinephrine and normal to slightly increased urine epinephrine, because these extra-adrenal neoplasms that behave otherwise as classic pheochromocytomas lack the phenylethanolamine-N-methyltransferase enzyme.

An abdominal CT with 3 mm cuts ("thin cuts") remains the current gold standard for localizing pheochromocytoma. Neoplasms that cause symptoms and/or signs are typically at least 2–3 cm in size. It is very important to image the entire abdomen to look for extra-adrenal pheochromocytomas and paragangliomas. Magnetic resonance imaging (MRI) can be used to both help confirm the diagnosis and localize the neoplasm. Pheochromocytomas are enhanced characteristically on T2-weighted images. MIBG scans take advantage of the fact that MIBG is incorporated selectively into adrenergic vesicles in pheochromocytomas. MIBG scanning is most valuable in looking for metastatic pheochromocytomas or extra-adrenal neoplasms. While MIBG scan is a good means of locating pheochromocytomas physiologically, the anatomic resolution is not precise and the test is only 90% sensitive.

Most pheochromocytomas, even large ones, can be removed laparoscopically depending on the surgeon's facility with the technique. Before resecting a pheochromocytoma, the patient must be prepared carefully with alpha-adrenergic blockade for at least one week. We prefer phenoxybenzamine, because it works well and is easy to titrate in an outpatient setting. Starting at 10 mg twice a day, the phenoxybenzamine is increased every few days until the patient is relatively normotensive and somewhat symptomatic (i.e., slight orthostatic hypotension, stuffy nose, decreased energy, etc); some patients may require up to a total of 200–300 mg a day. As the oral alpha-blockade proceeds, the catecholamine-induced volume contraction relaxes, the patient gains weight, and the hematocrit decreases. Other medications, such as prazosin, doxazosin, and calcium-channel blockers, can also be used for alpha-blockade. If the patient remains or becomes tachycardic after adequate alpha-blockade, a beta-blocker is added. Beta-blockers are most useful for patients with pre-existing cardiac disease. It is critically important that adequate alpha-blockade precede beta-blockade, because unopposed alpha-mediated vasoconstriction may lead to worsening hypertension, congestive heart failure, and cardiovascular collapse. During the operation, the patient should have an arterial catheter for continuous blood pressure monitoring and a large-bore peripheral or central venous catheter for drug and fluid infusion. The anesthesiologist should be prepared for wide fluctuations in blood pressure and heart rate. Medications, such as sodium nitroprusside, esmolol, ephedrine, and phenylephrine, should be readily available at all times during the operation. With adequate pre-operative alpha-blockade, patients usually do not have hemodynamic problems.

Aldosteronoma

About 1% of all patients with hypertension will have primary hyperaldosteronism (Fig. 6.2). Half of the patients with primary hyperaldosteronism have unilateral adenoma and half have bilateral hyperplasia. Unilateral primary hyperplasia and adrenocortical cancer are rare. Differentiating between bilateral hyperplasia and unilateral adenoma is crucial, because only patients with unilateral adenoma would benefit from adrenalectomy. Classically, primary hyperaldosteronism or Conn's Syndrome is characterized by hypertension refractory to medical therapy, hypokalemia, and polyuria. Patients may also present with muscle weakness, polydipsia, headaches, fatigue, hypernatremia, and a hypochloremic

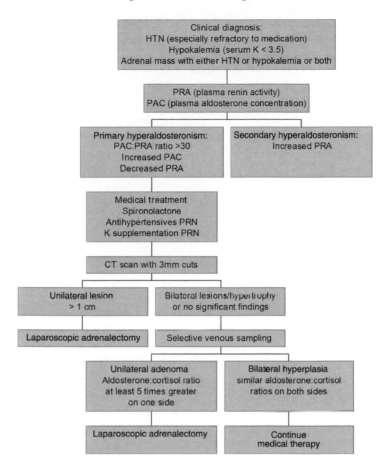

FIGURE 6.2. Work-up for aldosteronoma.

metabolic alkalosis. Patients with a unilateral adenoma tend to be younger, have more severe hypertension and hypokalemia (<3.0 mEq/l), and have higher urine and plasma aldosterone concentrations (>25ng/dl) than patients with bilateral hyperplasia. The diagnosis of primary hyperaldosteronism is made by an increased plasma aldosterone concentration (PAC), low plasma renin activity (PRA), and a PAC:PRA ratio > 20–30. Excess aldosterone suppresses renin secretion. An increased PAC (>5 ng/dl) or urinary aldosterone secretion (> 12 ng/dl) after 2l of saline infusion over four hours confirms the diagnosis in equivocal cases. With the increasing sensitivity of CT, postural stimulation tests and NP-59 scans are seldom utilized.

Abdominal CT with thin cuts (3 mm) through the adrenal glands is the best means of distinguishing an adenoma from bilateral hyperplasia. Clinically active aldosteronomas are typically hypodense and measure between 0.5 and 2 cm in size. Diminutive neoplasms (<0.5 cm) and micronodular hyperplasia may be mistaken for bilateral hyperplasia. Although some surgeons use selective venous sampling routinely to distinguish adenoma from hyperplasia, we only use venous sampling in about 20% of our patients in whom the CT shows bilateral abnormality or no abnormality of the adrenal glands.

The standard selective venous catheterization protocol, either with or without ACTH stimulation, entails drawing blood samples for cortisol and aldosterone from both adrenal veins and the inferior vena cava. The goals of selective venous catheterization are to (1) cannulate both adrenal veins, and (2) attempt to lateralize the tumor. Because the right adrenal vein is usually a short branch directly off the vena cava, it is often difficult to cannulate; the failure rate varies from 5% to 30% depending on the experience of the radiologist. An adrenal vein:inferior vena cava cortisol ratio of less than 3:1 signifies that the adrenal vein was not successfully cannulated and that the results are unreliable. A ratio greater than 3:1 indicates a successful cannulation. Unilateral aldosteronoma is confirmed if the adrenal vein aldosterone:cortisol ratio is at least five times higher on one side (see Fig. 6.3.). Aldosterone to cortisol ratios less than 5:1 suggest bilateral hyperplasia and medical management with spironolactone is indicated. Bilateral adrenalectomy is not indicated for bilateral hyperplasia, because it causes hypocortisolism (Addison's disease).

The treatment for an aldosteronoma is laparoscopic adrenalectomy. Patients are usually started on spironolactone, a competitive inhibitor of aldosterone, to control hypertension and hypokalemia pre-operatively. Other

Selective venous sampling for primary hyperaldosteronism
Name/date:

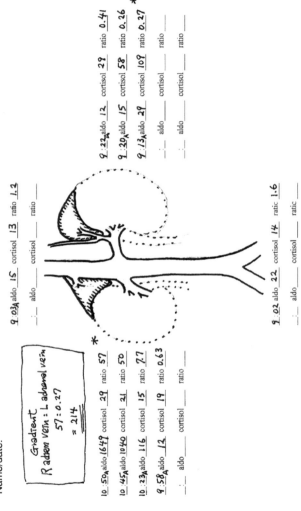

Figure 6.3. Tabulated results of selective venous sampling for primary hyperaldosteronism with a clear elevation in the aldosterone to cortisol ratio.

anti-hypertensives and potassium supplements are added as needed. Over 95% of patients become normokalemic immediately after adrenalectomy. Adrenalectomy corrects or improves hypertension in 75% of patients within one month of operation. Half of responders will be off all anti-hypertensives and half will require fewer medications than pre-operatively. For patients with an adenoma, it is important to stop spironolactone and potassium supplementation after the operation. Recurrence is rare.

Adrenal Cushing's Syndrome

Cushing's syndrome (see Fig. 6.4.) is caused by glucocorticoid excess and characterized by central obesity (90%), hypertension (85%), moonfaces, easy bruisability, skin changes (purple striae, hirsutism, acne, plethora), weakness, depression, polyuria, and glucose intolerance or diabetes. Exogenous steroid use is the most common cause of Cushing's syndrome. Endogenous glucocorticoid hypersecretion can be divided into ACTH-dependent and ACTH-independent causes. ACTH-dependent neoplasms overproduce ACTH and comprise 80% of endogenous Cushing's syndrome. Most of such patients have pituitary adenomas/hyperplasia (a.k.a. Cushing's disease), but some have ectopic, non-adrenal ACTH-secreting neoplasms (small cell lung cancer, bronchial carcinoids, thymomas, and pancreatic islet cell neoplasms). ACTH overproduction stimulates bilateral adrenal hyperplasia and glucocorticoid excess. ACTH-independent neoplasms (a.k.a. adrenal Cushing's syndrome) are caused by adrenocortical adenomas, adrenocortical carcinomas, or macro-or micronodular hyperplasia. The evaluation for Cushing's syndrome revolves around confirming the diagnosis and differentiating between ACTH-dependent and -independent neoplasms.

Nearly all patients with glucocorticoid hypersecretion lose normal hypothalamic control of cortisol secretion, as evidenced by the loss of diurnal variation of plasma cortisol concentrations. An increased 24-h urine-free cortisol secretion

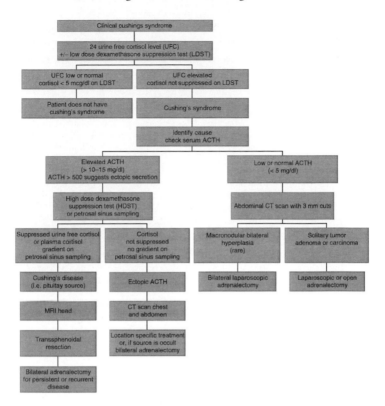

FIGURE 6.4. Cushing's syndrome.

is very sensitive and specific (95%) for the diagnosis of Cushing's syndrome. The diagnosis may be confirmed by a failure to suppress plasma cortisol concentrations after overnight, low-dose dexamethasone suppression testing. Increased midnight salivary cortisol level can also confirm Cushing's syndrome. After making the diagnosis of hypercortisolism, measuring plasma ACTH levels will differentiate between ACTH-dependent and ACTH-independent Cushing's syndrome. Low ACTH levels (<5 pg/ml) signify an ACTH-independent neoplasm (excess cortisol suppresses the release of ACTH by the pituitary). In contrast, an increased plasma ACTH level (>15 pg/ml) indicates lack of feedback inhibition and therefore an autonomous ACTH-producing neoplasm. The high dose dexamethasone suppression test is used to further distinguish between a pituitary and ectopic source of ACTH (pituitary neoplasms suppress), whereas ectopic ACTH-producing neoplasms do not. Furthermore, a very high plasma ACTH level (greater than 500 pg/ml) usually signifies an ectopic ACTH-producing lesion. The most specific test to distinguish pituitary from ectopic source of ACTH is petrosal sinus sampling for ACTH level after corticotropin-releasing hormone (CRH) stimulation.

CT and MRI may confirm the site of pathology and direct treatment. Pituitary adenomas seen on MRI with gadolinium contrast and thin cuts through the sellar region are either resected transsphenoidally or irradiated if the patient is a poor surgical candidate. Bilateral adrenalectomy can be curative for recurrent or persistent Cushing's disease if treatment directed against the pituitary fails. CT of the chest and abdomen (with thin cuts through the pancreas) may identify the location of ectopic ACTH-producing neoplasms. Patients with an occult source of ACTH should also be treated with laparoscopic bilateral adrenalectomy. For suspected adrenal Cushing's syndrome (ACTH-independent Cushing's), an abdominal CT with thin cuts through the adrenal bed will identify the adenoma or carcinoma and very rarely macronodular bilateral hyperplasia.

Because the contralateral normal adrenal gland is often suppressed in patients with adrenal Cushing's syndrome, patients should receive stress dose steroids perioperatively (hydrocortisone 100 mg IV Q 6 h).The steroids are tapered to an oral regimen in the post-operative period as clinically indicated (prednisone 20 mg in the morning and 10 mg in the evening). These patients are also more prone to infection and should receive one perioperative dose of antibiotics. While the majority of adrenal Cushing's syndrome is caused by adenomas, adrenocortical cancers may also secrete cortisol. Therefore, the surgeon should have a low threshold for converting laparoscopic adrenalectomy to an open procedure if evidence of malignancy is found. Patients who undergo bilateral laparoscopic adrenalectomy for bilateral hyperplasia (caused by ACTH-dependent Cushing's or nodular hyperplasia) require lifetime glucocorticoid and mineral corticoid (Florinef 0.1 mg/day) replacement.

Virilizing and Feminizing Neoplasms

Virilizing and feminizing adrenal neoplasms are distinctly uncommon. Because these neoplasms are rare and usually symptomatic, sex steroid levels should be checked only if there is evidence of virilization or feminization. Unfortunately, almost all feminizing neoplasms and half of virilizing neoplasms are adrenocortical cancers. Women with hirsutism, irregular menses, and other virilizing signs may have a hypersecreting adrenal neoplasm, congenital adrenal hyperplasia, or cystic ovarian disease. Increased levels of serum testosterone, serum dihydroepiandrostenedione (DHEA), and 24-h urine 17-hydroxy and ketosteroids establish the diagnosis of a virilizing neoplasm. Men with gynecomastia, impotence, loss of libido, or testicular atrophy may have a hypersecreting adrenal neoplasm or testicular neoplasm. Increased serum estrogen and suppressed serum FSH, LH, and gonadotropins confirm the diagnosis of a feminizing neoplasm. CT of the abdomen will confirm the presence of an adrenal neoplasm. For small virilizing adrenal neoplasms with no malignant features on CT, a laparoscopic approach may be attempted as long as the surgeon has a low threshold for conversion to open resection.

Adrenocortical Carcinoma

Adrenocortical cancer (ACC) is a rare neoplasm with a yearly incidence of 1 per million people in the United States. The median age at diagnosis is 40–50 years old with a 2:1 female-to-male ratio. Up to 80% of ACCs are functional (30% secrete cortisol, 20% androgens, 10% estrogen, 35% mixed hormones, and 1% aldosterone). The remaining neoplasms are non-functioning and are usually diagnosed as a large symptomatic mass. Rarely, small adrenocortical cancers can present as incidentalomas, but the vast majority of ACCs are usually large at the time of presentation, averaging 12–16 cm. An adrenal mass greater than 6 cm has about a 25% risk for malignancy. At the time of resection, one third of patients with cortical carcinoma will have localized disease, one third have regional disease, and one third have metastatic disease.

The surgeon should suspect cancer when dealing with a tumor that secretes cortisol, androgens, and/or estrogen. In particular, tumors that secrete multiple hormones are more likely to be malignant. On CT, adrenocortical cancers tend to be heterogeneous with irregular borders and areas of hemorrhage or necrosis. Tumors with a Hounsfield unit greater than 20 are likely to be malignant. The CT should be reviewed for signs of invasion into adjacent structures and organs or renal veins or vena cava, as well as for regional lymphadenopathy and metastases. The most common sites for metastatic disease include the liver, lung, peritoneum, and bones. Because gadolinium accumulates and persists in malignancies, MRI can demonstrate the presence or absence of vascular invasion. Tumor thrombus in the inferior vena cava is considered regional disease and should be resected using veno-venous bypass if needed.

En bloc resection of adrenocortical cancer, involved structures, and retroperitoneal fat is the only chance for cure. Open adrenalectomy is indicated to ensure complete resection and avoid tumor rupture. With adequate resection, the 5-year survivals for patients with stage I and II neoplasms are 40–60%. For stage III disease (potentially resectable local invasion or nodes), the 5-year survival decreases to 20–30% even with complete resection. Only 10% of patients with stage IV disease (metastases, unresectable local organ invasion) survive past 1 year. Significant palliation may be achieved in patients with functional or symptomatic tumors. Up to 85% of patients will develop recurrent or metastatic disease. Mitotane is the most common adjuvant therapy for patients with residual, recurrent, or metastatic disease; unfortunately, it has a low remission rate (20–35%) and significant

GI and neurologic side effects. In contrast, mitotane is effective for palliation with 80% of patients demonstrating a decrease in hypersecretion.

Adrenal Metastases

An adrenal mass in a patient with a history of cancer should be suspected of being a metastasis, especially if the mass is over 4 cm. Up to 75% of such lesions are metastases. In contrast, in a patient without a concurrent diagnosis of cancer or a history of cancer, an adrenal mass is almost never a metastasis. Lung cancer (especially small cell and adenocarcinoma), renal cell carcinoma, melanoma, gastrointestinal cancer, breast cancer, lymphoma, and hepatocellular carcinoma are the most common metastases to the adrenal gland. Finding multiple synchronous metastases is a more common scenario than finding a single adrenal metastasis. Unfortunately, patients with multiple lesions have a worse prognosis.

Bone or abdominal pain, weight loss, night sweats, hemoptysis, constipation, and early satiety are all symptoms suggestive of metastatic disease. Patients with a solitary adrenal lesion should have screening appropriate for age and risk factors, such as colonoscopy, mammography, and chest x-ray, to identify possible primary cancer. On CT, bilateral lesions, large tumors, irregular borders, local invasion, hemorrhage, and tumor necrosis suggest malignancy. Positron emission tomography (PET) can support the diagnosis of cancer and identify other metastatic foci. Fine needle aspiration may confirm the diagnosis but should only be performed after a pheochromocytoma has been definitively excluded. Inadvertent biopsy of a pheochromocytoma is potentially lethal.

A patient with widely metastatic disease is not a candidate for resection. In contrast, resection may be curative for patients with solitary metastasis. The longer the disease-free interval between initial resection of the primary cancer and discovery of the metachronous adrenal metastasis, the better the prognosis. As with adrenocortical cancers, complete en bloc resection must be performed. Fortunately, isolated adrenal metastases are often encapsulated within the adrenal gland and easily removed. Laparoscopic adrenalectomy is as safe and effective as open resection. Systemic recurrence is a problem, but local recurrence is rare. After adrenalectomy, the five-year survival is 25% with a mean survival ranging from 20–30 months in contrast to 6–8 months without resection.

Incidentaloma

Incidentaloma (see Fig. 6.5.) is as an adrenal tumor discovered on diagnostic imaging done for non-adrenal disorders. Incidentalomas has become more common with the improved resolution and more widespread use of imaging techniques. The prevalence of incidentalomas is estimated to be 1–4% of abdominal imaging studies and increases with increasing age of the study cohort. Most incidentalomas are non-functioning adenomas and require no treatment. The main reasons for resecting incidentaloma are hormone hypersecretion and a high risk of cancer. Currently about one-third of pheochromocytomas and adrenal Cushing's neoplasm present as incidentalomas and are only diagnosed after appropriate biochemical testing. Most surgeons advise resection for all functional tumors and all tumors larger than 5–6 cm. About 5% of non-functioning 3–5 cm lesions are cancers. In this group, tumor size, patient preference, age, and co-morbidities should be considered when deciding whether or not to recommend adrenalectomy. Unless there is clear evidence of malignancy, these tumors maybe resected laparoscopically and can be converted to an open or hand-assisted operation if malignant features are found intra-operatively or a complete laparoscopic resection cannot be performed. Ninety percent of incidentalomas are smaller than 2 cm. Tumors smaller than 3 cm and those that are 3–5 cm but treated non-operatively may be followed with repeat abdominal imaging every 6 months to a year and with yearly screening for cortisol and catecholamine hypersecretion. Twenty-five percent of incidentalomas will grow, and 20% will hypersecrete over a 10-year follow-up period.

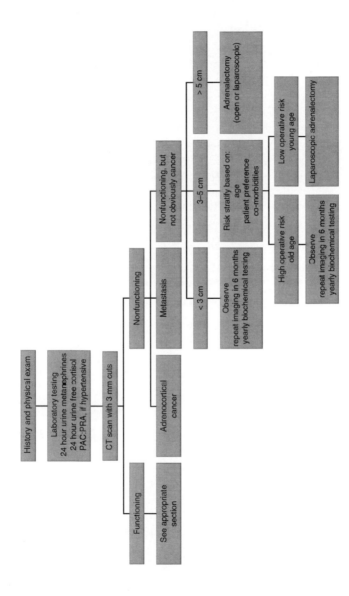

FIGURE 6.5. Work-up for incidentaloma.

Conclusion

Adrenal tumors are a diverse group. The primary goals during workup are to determine if it is functional and if it is a cancer. Hypersecreting tumors and tumors suspicious for malignancy should be resected.

In the past 10 years, laparoscopic adrenalectomy has become the standard of care for treating most adrenal tumors. Multiple, non-randomized trials have demonstrated that patients have less pain, shorter recovery times, and fewer complications after laparoscopic adrenalectomy when compared to open resection. Most adrenal tumors can be resected laparoscopically by experience surgeons. Patients with very large(>10–12 cm) tumors or obviously invasive adrenocortical carcinomas should have open resection.

Selected Readings

Brunt LM, et al. (2001) Outcomes analysis in patients undergoing laparoscopic adrenalectomy for hormonally active adrenal tumors. Surgery 130:629

Grumbach M, Biller B, Braunstein G, et al. (2003) Management of the clinically inapparent adrenal mass. Ann Intern Med 138:424

Lal G, Duh QY (2003) Laparoscopic adrenalectomy - indications and technique. Surg Oncol 12:105–123

Liao CH, Chueh SC, Lai MK, et al. (2006) Laparoscopic adrenalectomy for potentially malignant adrenal tumors greater than 5 cm. J Clin Endocrinol Metabol 91:3080–3083

Shen WT, Sturgeon C, Duh QY (2005) From incidentaloma to adrenocortical carcinoma: the surgical management of adrenal tumors. J Surg Oncol 89:186–192

7

Neuroendocrine Tumors of the Pancreas

Volker Fendrich and Matthias Rothmund

Pearls and Pitfalls

Insulinomas

- 90% are single, benign, small tumors of the pancreas.
- Do not rely on preoperative imaging procedures.
- Exclude factitious hypoglycemia.
- Enucleation is procedure of choice.
- Avoid blind distal pancreatic resection.
- Malignancy can only be proven by angioinvasion and metastases.
- Aggressive treatment of metastatic insulinomas is recommended.
- Resection of the tumor is the only chance for cure.

Gastrinomas

- Most gastrinomas are located in the "gastrinoma triangle," comprising the head of the pancreas, and the first and second parts of the duodenum.
- 20% of gastrinomas occur within the MEN1-syndrome.
- 50–60% of tumors are malignant at the time of diagnosis.
- Duodenotomy is an essential part of the operation.
- Only patients with complete tumor resection have 5-and 10-year survival rates of 90%.
- Biochemical evidence justifies operation.
- Pylorus-preserving pancreaticoduodenectomy may be the procedure of choice for MEN1-ZES.

K.I. Bland et al. (eds.), *Endocrine Surgery*,
DOI: 10.1007/978-1-84996-447-0_7,
© Springer-Verlag London Limited 2011

Non-functioning Tumors

- Symptoms may mimic those of pancreatic carcinoma.
- 60–90% malignancy rate.
- An aggressive surgical approach is justified even for patients with metastases.
- Most common tumor present in MEN1 patients.
- Resect if > 1 cm in size.

Introduction

Pancreaticoduodenal endocrine tumors (PETs) represent an important subset of pancreatic neoplasms (Table 7.1.) and for 2–4% of all clinically detected pancreatic tumors. They consist of single or multiple, benign or malignant neoplasms, and in 10–20%, are associated with multiple endocrine neoplasia type 1 (MEN1). PETs present as either functional tumors, causing specific hormonal syndromes, such as Zollinger-Ellison syndrome and organic hyperinsulinism, or as non-functional tumors with symptoms similar to those associated with pancreatic adenocarcinoma. This chapter focuses on these three tumors, as they represent 90% of all PETs. Special aspects of patients with MEN1-PETs will also be described. An algorithm for clinical management of PETs is indicated in Fig. 7.1.

Insulinomas

Insulinomas are the most frequent of all functional PETs. The incidence is reportedly 2–4 patients per million population per year. Insulinomas have been diagnosed in all age groups with the highest incidence between 40–60 years. Females seem to be slightly more frequently affected. The etiology and pathogenesis of insulinomas are unknown. No risk factors have been associated with these tumors. Virtually all insulinomas are located in the pancreas or are directly attached to it. Tumors are equally distributed within the

TABLE 7.1. Neuroendocrine tumors of the pancreas.

Tumor (Syndrome)	Incidence	Presentation	Malignancy
Insulinoma	70–80%	Weakness, sweating, tremulousness, tachycardia, anxiety, fatigue, headache, dizziness, disorientation, seizures, and unconsciousness	<10%
Gastrinoma	20–25%	Intractable or recurrent peptic ulcer disease (hemorrhage, perforation), complications of peptic ulcer, diarrhea	50–60%
Non-functional tumors	30–50%	Obstructive jaundice, pancreatitis, epigastric pain, duodenal obstruction, weight loss, fatigue	60–90%
VIPoma	4%	Profuse watery diarrhea, hypotension, abdominal pain	80%
Glucagonoma	4%	Migratory, necrolytic skin rash, glossitis, stomatitis, angular cheilitis, diabetes, severe weight loss, diarrhea	80%
Somatostatinoma	<5%	Weight loss, cholelithiasis, diarrhea, neurofibromatosis	50%
Carcinoid	<1%	Flushing, sweating, diarrhea, edema, wheezing	90%
ACTHoma	<1%	Cushing's syndrome	>90%
GRFoma	<1%	Acromegaly	30%
PTH-like-oma	<1%	Hypercalcemia, bone pain	>90%
Neurotensinoma	<1%	Hypotension, tachycardia, malabsorption	>80%

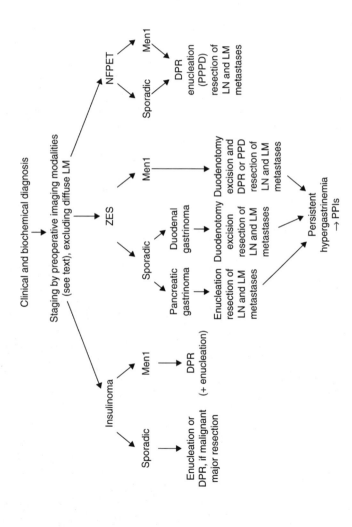

FIGURE 7.1. Algorithm of clinical management of PETs. ZES: Zollinger-Ellison syndrome; NFPET: non-functioning endocrine tumors of the pancreas; LM: liver metastases; LN: lymph node metastases; PPPD: pylorus-preserving pancreaticoduodenectomy; PPI: proton pump inhibitors.

gland. Approximately 90% of insulinomas are solitary; about 10% are multiple and are associated with MEN1-syndrome.

Prognosis and Predictive Factors

No immunohistochemical markers are available which reliably predict the biological behavior of insulinoma. The incidence of malignant insulinomas is about 10%. Insulinomas of <2 cm in diameter without signs of angioinvasion or metastases are considered benign.

Clinical Symptoms

Insulinomas are characterized by fasting hypoglycemia and neuroglycopenic symptoms, and occasionally by sympathoadrenal autonomic symptoms. The episodic nature of the hypoglycemic attacks is due to the intermittent insulin secretion by the tumor. The severity of symptoms does not always predict malignancy or the size of the tumor. The most important symptoms of central nervous system dysfunction include diplopia, blurred vision, confusion, abnormal behavior, and amnesia. Some patients develop loss of consciousness, coma, or even permanent brain damage. The release of catecholamines produces symptoms such as sweating, weakness, hunger, tremor, nausea, anxiety, and palpitation. The diagnosis is suspected with Whipple's triad, i.e. symptoms of hypoglycemia, plasma glucose levels <30 mg/dl, and relief of symptoms on intravenous administration of glucose.

Diagnostic Procedures

Biochemical Testing

A fasting test that may last up to 72 h is regarded as the most sensitive test. Insulin, proinsulin, C-peptide, and blood glucose are measured in 1–2 h intervals to demonstrate an inappropriately high secretion of insulin in relation to blood glucose. About

80% of insulinomas are diagnosed by this test, most in the first 24 h. A continuous C-peptide level demonstrates the endogenous secretion of insulin and excludes factitious hypoglycemia by insulin injection. Other differential etiologies of hypoglycemia include hormonal deficiencies, hepatic insufficiency, medication, drugs, and enzyme defects. Occasionally, differentiating insulinoma from these other causes of hypoglycemia can be quite difficult. Nesidioblastosis is a rare disorder and require intraoperative biopsy to differentiate it from insulinoma. This pathologic entity is characterized by replacement of normal pancreatic islets by diffuse hyperplasia of islet cells.

Imaging

It is well known and accepted that intraoperative exploration of the pancreas is the best method to localize insulinomas. Our study of 40 patients with insulinomas has shown that the tumor was correctly localized before operation in 65% by endoscopic ultrasound (EU), 33% by computed tomography (CT) and abdominal ultrasound (US), 15% by magnetic resonance tomography (MRT), and 0% by somatostatin-receptor-scintigraphy (SRS). On the other hand, all tumors were identified and resected after surgical exploration and intraoperative ultrasound (IOUS) of the pancreas after extensive mobilization of the gland. We recommend US or CT scan to exclude malignant metastasizing insulinomas. For localization of an insulinoma, EU has the highest sensitivity. It should be used, especially if a laparoscopic resection is considered. If no lesion is identified, and one can rely on the biochemical tests for diagnosis, laparotomy should follow.

Treatment

Benign Insulinoma

Surgical cure rates in patients with the biochemical diagnosis of insulinoma range from 77% to 100%. At surgical exploration, the abdomen is initially explored for evidence of metastatic disease. Then a meticulous surgical exploration should follow, i.e. an extended Kocher maneuver to allow palpation of the head. Mobilization of the distal pancreas and the spleen should follow to explore the body and tail of the gland and examine the distal pancreas carefully and completely. IOUS should be used to confirm the presence of tumor, to find nonpalpable lesions, and also to observe the relation of the tumor to the pancreatic duct. Intraoperative palpation has been shown to be a reliable method for localizing insulinomas—with successful identification of near 100% of tumors. As the combination of palpation and IOUS is a very effective method of intraoperative tumor localization, invasive preoperative localization studies are not necessary, and used only for patients with persistent or recurrent disease. IOUS is also useful in determining the relationship of insulinomas to the pancreatic duct and major vessels. Identification of the pancreatic duct and determination of its proximity to the tumor can guide safe enucleation of the tumor. This approach can minimize the likelihood of a postoperative pancreatic fistula. Tumor enucleation, when feasible, is the technique of choice.

Postoperatively, blood sugar levels begin to rise in most patients within the first hours after removal of an insulinoma (reactive hyperglycemia). To preserve pancreatic function and reduce the risk of iatrogenic diabetes mellitus, patients in whom tumor localization is not successful at operation should not undergo blind resection. These patients should be carefully evaluated by an experienced endocrine surgeon for confirmation of the diagnosis and further treatment.

Recent advances in laparoscopic technique and instrumentation have enabled surgeons to approach complex procedures laparoscopically. This is also true for insulinomas. The pancreas is exposed after opening the lesser sac and mobilizing its head. Laparoscopic ultrasound can be used to identify nonvisible tumors and determine the relationship of the lesion to surrounding veins and the pancreatic duct. Laparoscopic ultrasound can be particularly helpful in identifying lesions in

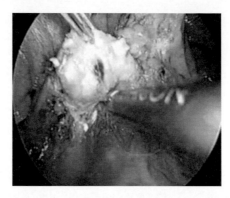

FIGURE 7.2. Laparoscopic enucleation of a ventral insulinoma.

the tail that are often missed by endoscopic ultrasound. For superficial ventral tumors, laparoscopic enucleation is undertaken with electrocautery or laparoscopic coagulating shears (Fig. 7.2). Small pancreatic vessels can be clipped and cut. Tumors located deep in the body or tail of the pancreas and those in close proximity to the pancreatic duct require distal pancreatectomy. In cases where visualization and ultrasound fail, a hand port can be used to allow palpation of the gland. Tumors situated very distally near the splenic hilum are especially difficult to identify. Spleen-sparing distal pancreatectomy can be accomplished by careful division of the short gastric vessels and stapling of the pancreas.

Malignant Insulinoma

These tumors must show evidence of either local invasion into surrounding soft tissue or verification of lymph node or liver metastasis to be considered malignant. Malignant insulinomas account for only about 5–10% of all insulinomas. Aggressive attempts at resection are recommended as these tumors are much less virulent than their malignant ductal exocrine counterparts. Also, there is no effective medical treatment available. The ten-year survival rate of 29% has been reported in malignant insulinomas. When surgical options to treat malignant insulinomas cannot be applied or have been exhausted, radiofrequency ablation is utilized for palliation. Chemotherapeutic options include Adriamycin and streptozocin which have achieved a 69% tumor regression rate, and remission from endocrine symptoms has extended to 18 months. Unfortunately, because this combination of drugs is also associated with considerable toxicity, it is usually reserved for patients only when they develop symptoms and no other options are available.

MEN1 Insulinomas

Since there is no good medical option to adequately control the symptoms of hormonal excess, surgical resection is generally recommended, even if no tumor is detectable by preoperative imaging, as long as diffuse metastatic disease is excluded. We recommend distal pancreatic resection to the level of the portal vein with preservation of the spleen and enucleation of PETs of the pancreatic head in the case of multiple tumors, or enucleation in the case of a single PET. The reported cure rates of this approach for MEN1-associated organic hyperinsulinism are excellent. In our own patient population, all six MEN1 patients with organic hyperinsulinism are cured after a median follow-up of 88 months.

Gastrinomas (Zollinger-Ellison-Syndrome)

Gastrinomas are relatively common, functionally active endocrine tumors of the pancreas, accounting for about 20% of cases, second in frequency to insulinomas. Approximately 0.1% of patients with duodenal ulcers have evidence of Zollinger-Ellison syndrome (ZES). The reported incidence is between 0.5 and4 per million per year. ZES is more common in males than in females, with a ratio of 3:2. The mean age at the onset of symptoms is 38 years, range 7–83 years in some series. The etiology and pathogenesis of sporadic gastrinomas are unknown. Approximately 20% of gastrinomas are part of MEN-1. No other risk factors are known. At the time of diagnosis, 50–60% of tumors are malignant. Pancreatic gastrinomas occur more frequently in the head of the pancreas. More than 90% of the duodenal gastrinomas are located in the first and second part of the duodenum, and are limited to the submucosa in 54% of patients. The anatomical area comprising the head of the pancreas, the superior and descending portion of the duodenum, and the relevant lymph nodes has been called the "gastrinoma triangle", since it harbors the vast majority of these tumors.

Prognosis and Predictive Factors

In general, the progression of gastrinomas is relatively slow with a combined 5-year survival rate of 65% and 10-year survival rate of 51%. Patients with complete tumor resection have excellent 5- and 10-year survival rates (90–100%). Patients with pancreatic tumors have a worse prognosis than those with primary tumors in the duodenum. There is no established marker to predict the biological behavior of gastrinoma.

Clinical Symptoms

Over 90% of patients with gastrinomas have peptic ulcer disease, with multiple ulcers sometimes at unusual sites. Diarrhea is another common symptom caused by the large volume of gastric acid secretion. The low pH inactivates pancreatic enzymes, leading to malabsorption and steatorrhea. Abdominal pain from either peptic ulcer disease or gastroesophageal reflux disease remains the most common symptom, occurring in more than 75% of patients.

Diagnostic Procedures

Biochemical Testing

If the patient presents with gastric pH below 2.5 and serum gastrin concentration above 1,000 pg/ml (normal <100 pg/ml), then the diagnosis of Zollinger-Ellison is confirmed. Unfortunately, many (40–50%) patients present with serum gastrin concentrations between 100 and 500 pg/ml, and in these patients a secretin test should be performed. The secretin test is considered positive when an increase in serum gastrin over the pre-treatment value is >200 pg/ml, together with a low pH in the stomach. The clinical picture and a secretin test rule out gastrinoma versus other causes of hypergastrinemia (e.g. atrophic gastritis).

Imaging

The size of gastrinomas varies with the site of the tumors: pancreatic gastrinomas are often larger than 1 cm, whereas gastrinomas of the duodenum are usually smaller than 1 cm in diameter. Therefore, it is nearly impossible to identify duodenal gastrinomas by preoperative imaging procedures. In a recent study in patients with sporadic ZES, gastrinomas were detected by US in 24%, by CT in 39%, by MRI in 46%, and by selective angiography in 48%. In approximately one-third of patients with sporadic gastrinomas, the results of conventional imaging studies were negative. A European multicenter trial to evaluate the efficacy of somatostatin-receptor-scintigraphy (SRS) showed positive results in pancreatic gastrinomas in 73%. As in insulinomas, the best methods to localize gastrinomas are surgical exploration, IOUS, and duodenotomy. The sensitivities of palpation and IOUS are 91% and 95%, respectively, for pancreatic gastrinomas. On the basis of recent studies and our own experience, we recommend using either US or CT and SRS before primary operations, primarily for staging of the disease. This should be followed by exploratory laparotomy including duodenotomy and complete mobilization of the pancreas followed by IOUS. For reoperative cases, ES and the selective arterial secretin injection test (Imamura technique) should be used to localize or regionalize solitary or multiple tumors.

Treatment

In 1999, a prospective study was published that involved 123 sporadic gastrinoma patients who had surgical resection of tumor and were assessed for 8 years postoperatively. In ninety-three percent of patients, gastrinoma was found, including each of the last 81 consecutive cases. The immediate postoperative cure rate was 60%, 40% at 5 years, and 34% at 10 years. Surgery was both safe and produced long-term cures in most patients. The *current surgical strategy for treatment of ZES* should include a thorough exploration and IOUS of the pancreas and longitudinal duodenotomy with separate palpation of the anterior and posterior walls to detect duodenal microgastrinomas. If diffuse metastases in both liver lobes are excluded, gastrinomas in the head of the pancreas should be enucleated and duodenal gastrinomas should be excised. A systematic sampling of all anterior and posterior lymph nodes around the head of the pancreas, the celiac axis, and the common bile duct must be performed, even if the lymph nodes appear macroscopically normal. Liver metastases are the most important prognostic factor in gastrinomas. They should be aggressively resected. Using this approach, we and others achieved 10-year survival rates of up to 100% in patients with malignant gastrinomas without distant metastases at the initial operation.

MEN1 Gastrinomas

MEN1 gastrinomas occur mainly in the duodenum. In the past they have been locally excised or treated by additional distal pancreatectomy. As liver metastases are the most important prognostic factor in MEN1-ZES, we have advocated a more aggressive surgical strategy. To avoid their recurrence, we recommend duodenopancreatic resections in MEN1 patients who have biochemical evidence of ZES. This aggressive surgical approach based on predictive genetic testing and regular surveillance not only prevents the development of liver metastases; it might also result in a higher cure rate of MEN1-ZES, since the tumors and their lymph node metastases are resected at the earliest possible stage. None of our 11 ZES patients developed postoperative liver metastases and 55% (7 of 11) had a negative secretin test after a median follow-up of 104 months. Another reason for these results might be the introduction of pylorus-preserving pancreaticoduodenectomy as the first-line procedure, if the gastrin source has been regionalized to the pancreatic head preoperatively. The rationale for this approach is that more than 90% of gastrinomas occur in the duodenum and thus, recurrence is impossible, if the organ of origin is removed.

Non-Functioning Tumors

Endocrine tumors of the pancreas are clinically classified as non-functional or non-functioning when they are not related to any definite clinical syndrome. They are most often diagnosed in the 5–6th decades of life. Nonfunctional pancreatic endocrine tumors (NFPETs) have increased in frequency compared to functional tumors and now represent 30–50% of PETs. Differentiation from the more aggressive pancreatic adenocarcinomas is extremely important (Table 7.2).

Prognosis and Predictive Factors

About 70% of all NFPETs are malignant. Overall 5- and 10-year survival rates of 65% and 49%, respectively, have been described. When comparing nonfunctioning with functioning pancreatic endocrine neoplasms, the non-functioning neoplasms seem to have a poorer prognosis.

TABLE 7.2. Differences between pancreatic cancer and non-functioning endocrine tumors of the pancreas (NFPET).

	Pancreatic cancer	NFPET
Tumor size	<5 cm	>5 cm
CT scan	Hypodensity; No calcifications	Hyperdensity; Calcifications possible
Chromogranin A in blood	Negative	Positive
Somatostatin-Receptor-Scintigraphy	Negative	Positive

Clinical Symptoms

Patients usually present late, owing to the lack of a clinical/hormonal marker of the tumor's activity. Therefore, in contrast to functioning PETs, patients with NFPETs present with various nonspecific symptoms, sometimes jaundice, distant metastases, or invasion of surrounding structures. Symptoms include abdominal pain, weight loss, and pancreatitis. The frequency of jaundice at presentation is higher in series with the tumor located in the pancreatic head. In some cases, liver metastases are the first symptom or finding.

Diagnostic Procedures

Biochemical Testing

There are general tumor markers, the most interesting being chromogranin A and pancreatic polypeptide (PP). Increased levels of chromogranin A have been reported in 50–80% of PETs and sometimes correlate with the tumor burden. The combination of chromogranin A with measurement of PP increased the sensitivity from 84% to 96% in non-functioning tumors.

Imaging

Preoperatively, US or CT scan are the procedures of choice and are usually effective, because these tumors are relatively large, usually more than 5 cm in diameter. SRS can be performed to differentiate endocrine from nonendocrine pancreatic tumors. Since almost all exocrine pancreatic carcinomas are SRS-negative, a positive SRS is highly suggestive for neuroendocrine carcinoma. Therefore, the potential value of SRS is primarily the determination of the tumor type and its extent, rather than its correct localization. Recognition of NFPETs is imperative because of their good resectability and excellent long-term survival compared to that of ductal pancreatic carcinoma.

Treatment

We advocate an aggressive surgical approach for the management of malignant non-functioning NFPETs even in the presence of localized metastases. The major goal is a potentially curative resection with no tumor tissue left behind. This may require partial pancreatoduodenectomy with resection and reconstruction of the superior mesenteric artery and/or the superior mesenteric-portal venous confluence, as well as the synchronous resection of liver metastases. Using an aggressive approach, potentially curative resections are possible in up to 62%, and overall 5-year survival rates around 65% can be achieved. Repeated resections for resectable recurrences or metastases are indicated in order to improve survival.

MEN1 NFPETs

There is very little data about the management of non-functional PETs in MEN1. There are several special facts and unresolved questions regarding this issue. Non-functional PETs are asymptomatic, often multiple, and occur in up to 85% of MEN1 patients as in our cohort of patients. The growth rate of non-functional PETs, as well as their meta-static potential, remains to be established. Metastatic spread even to distant sites has rarely been observed in small tumors (<2 cm in size). However, no distant metastases have yet developed in patients with NFPETs smaller than 1 cm in size. Therefore, we recommend an aggressive surgical approach to prevent the development of metastases, if the largest tumor size exceeds 10 mm on imaging. This includes distal pancreatic resection to the level of the portal vein and enucleation of PETs in the pancreatic head. In tumors of more than 2 cm in size or tumors with suspected malignancy in the distal pancreas, splenectomy should be performed to excise the lymph nodes from the splenic hilum, which is a frequent location of metastases. One must keep in mind that this strategy leads to long-term control of pancreatic disease in MEN1.

Selected Readings

Bartsch DK, Fendrich V, Langer P, et al. (2005) Outcome of duode-nopancreatic resections in patients with multiple endocrine neoplasia type 1. Ann Surg 242:757–764; discussion 764–766

Bartsch DK, Schilling T, Ramaswamy A, et al. (2000) Management of nonfunctioning islet cell carcinomas. World J Surg 24:1418–1424

Fendrich V, Bartsch DK, Langer P, et al. (2004) Diagnosis and therapy in 40 patients with insulinoma. Dtsch Med Wochenschr 129:941–946

Fendrich V, Bartsch DK, Langer P, et al. (2005) Zollinger-Ellison-Syndrome – the changing role of surgery. Chirurg 76:217–226

Fendrich V, Langer P, Celik I, et al. (2006) An aggressive surgical approach leads to long-term survival in patients with pancreatic endocrine tumors. Ann Surg 244:845–851

Norton JA, Fraker DL, Alexander HR, et al. (1999) Surgery to cure the Zollinger-Ellison syndrome. N Engl J Med 341:635–644

Thompson NW, Bondeson AG, Bondeson L, Vinik A (1989) The surgical treatment of gastrinoma in MENI syndrome patients. Surgery 106:1081

Van Heerden JA, Grant CS, Czako PF, Service FJ, Charboneau JW (1992) Occult functioning insulinomas: which localizing studies are indicated? Surgery 112:1010–1014

8

Carcinoid Neoplasms

Göran Åkerström and Per Hellman

Pearls and Pitfalls

Gastric Carcinoids

- Gastrin-dependent gastric carcinoids and gastric endocrine cell hyperplasia occur in 1% of patients with atrophic gastritis, and in MEN1 patients with Zollinger-Ellison syndrome, with increased gastric acid, and without mucosal atrophy.
- Correct diagnosis requires multiple gastric mucosal biopsies:
  - If biopsies show atrophic gastritis, the carcinoid is *type 1*; endoscopic excision and surveillance is adequate because risk for metastases is minimal.
  - If there is no atrophic gastritis and the patient has MEN1, the carcinoid is *type 2*, and usually single, larger, invasive, and requires resection.
  - In the absence of atrophic gastritis and MEN1, the lesion is *type 3*, sporadic gastric carcinoid prognosis is poorer, and aggressive resection is warranted.

Midgut Carcinoids

- The small ileal tumor and large mesenteric metastases encircled by fibrosis should raise suspicion of a midgut carcinoid.
- Even with grossly radical excision, liver metastases may occur after years of follow-up. Recurrence should

K.I. Bland et al. (eds.), *Endocrine Surgery*,
DOI: 10.1007/978-1-84996-447-0_8,
© Springer-Verlag London Limited 2011

be suspected with an increase in serum chromogranin A.

- Progressive mesenteric tumor fibrosis tends to entrap intestines and mesenteric vessels with resultant intestinal (venous) ischemia - prophylactic removal is indicated.
- Alleviation of the carcinoid syndrome may be achieved if large liver metastases are excised.
- Radiofrequency (RF) ablation widens indications for liver surgery for patients with bilateral metastases.

Appendiceal Carcinoids

- Appendiceal carcinoids are generally incidental and clinically insignificant.
- Tumors <2 cm without invasion or metastases are treated safely by appendectomy alone.
- Carcinoids >2 cm with invasion or lymph node metastases or any tumor in the base of the appendix requires right-sided hemicolectomy and lymph node clearance.
- Adeno-(goblet cell) carcinoids need aggressive surgical resection together with chemotherapy.

Colorectal Carcinoids

- Although cecal carcinoids are treated as midgut carcinoids and may cause the carcinoid syndrome, distal colon or rectal carcinoids do not manifest the carcinoid syndrome.
- The majority of rectal carcinoids are incidental, <1 cm, and are removed safely by endoscopy.
- Tumors of 1–2 cm are investigated by endosonography and are amenable to transanal resection provided there is no muscular invasion or regional lymphadenopathy.
- Tumors >2 cm or those with invasion or regional metastases are best treated by anterior resection and lymph node clearance.
- Virtually all patients with rectal carcinoids >2 cm develop distant metastases.

Carcinoids are rare neuroendocrine neoplasms with an incidence of 1–2 per 100,000 population per year; 70% occur in the gastrointestinal tract (Table 8.1). In a newer classification, the term "carcinoid tumors" depicts classical midgut carcinoid tumors, and other types of carcinoids are named neuroendocrine neoplasms of the respective organs. Neuroendocrine neoplasms are identified by chromogranin A and synaptophysin immunostains. The majority of carcinoid neoplasms are well differentiated (with low rate of mitoses and low Ki67 proliferation index, generally <2%), although some are intermediate or poorly differentiated with an increased rate of mitoses and higher proliferation index (with increased Ki67 index, 10–40%). The well-differentiated carcinoids generally have an extended disease course, and the specific indications for extended resection depend on tumor type and localization. The role of operative resection is less evident for the poorly differentiated lesions, some of which may respond to chemotherapy. Most neuroendocrine tumors are clinically non-functioning, but in some carcinoids, specific hormone secretion may cause typical clinical syndromes (Table 8.2), the most common of which is the carcinoid syndrome associated with the classic midgut carcinoid with multiple hepatic metastases.

TABLE 8.1. Distribution of carcinoid tumors by site (Data from Modlin et al., 2003).

Site	Occurrence (%)
Extra-gastrointestinal (lung, thymic, ovary, uterus)	33
Esophagus	<1
Stomach	4
Duodenum/pancreas	2
Small intestine	32
Appendix	8
Colon	10
Rectum	11

TABLE 8.2. Classification of carcinoid tumors, hormone production and syndromes (Adapted from Öberg, 1998).

Category	Localization	Hormone production	Syndrome
Foregut carcinoids	Thymus	ACTH, CRF	Ectopic Cushing's syndrome, acromegaly, atypical carcinoid syndrome
	Lung	ACTH, CRF, ADH, GRH, gastrin, PP, hCG-α/β, serotonin	
	Stomach	Gastrin, histamine (serotonin)	Atypical carcinoid syndrome
	Duodenum	Gastrin, somatostatin	Zollinger-Ellison syndrome
	Pancreas	(Serotonin)	(Carcinoid syndrome)
Midgut carcinoids	Jejunum-ileum	Serotonin, NKA	Classical carcinoid syndrome
	Proximal colon	Substance P, bradykinin, prostaglandins (serotonin)	(Carcinoid syndrome)
	Appendix	No hormone production	
Hindgut carcinoids	Colon	PYY	
	Rectum	hCG-α/β	

ACTH, adrenocorticotropic hormone; ADH, antidiuretic hormone (vasopressin); CRF, corticotropin-releasing factor; GRH, growth hormone; hCG, human choriogonadotropin (α/β subunits); NKA, neurokinin A; PP, pancreatic polypeptide; PYY, peptide YY.

Gastric Carcinoids

Gastric carcinoids are rare, constituting 1% of gastric neoplasms and 4% of all carcinoids.

Type 1 gastric carcinoids: The most common gastric carcinoids (70–80%) occur secondary to hypergastrinemia and are found most commonly in patients with autoimmune chronic atrophic gastritis (CAG) (Fig. 8.1). These carcinoids are typically multicentric, develop concomitant with enterochromaffin-like (ECL) cell hyperplasia in the gastric body and fundus, and occur most commonly in older female patients at a mean age of about 65 years. These types of carcinoid neoplasms occur in CAG-induced atrophic fundic mucosa secondary to the hypergastrinemia caused by the absence of gastric acid secretion.

Typically, these carcinoids appear as multiple, small gastric polyps and are associated invariably with ECL cell hyperplasia in the surrounding gastric mucosa. The number of gross lesions varies, though some tumors appear solitary. Carcinoid polyps may be difficult to distinguish from adenomatous polyps, which are also common in CAG patients. Only a few ever ulcerate or bleed. The majority are benign without invasion beyond the submucosa into the muscularis propria. These CAG-associated carcinoids have a very low incidence of metastases to regional lymph glands (<5%) or distant metastases(<2%), and disease-related deaths are very rare indeed. The carcinoids up to 1 cm are indolent with minimal risk for invasion and can be treated by endoscopic mucosectomy if histology excludes deep gastric wall invasion. Local operative excision is recommended for the rare larger or invasive neoplasms; exceptional patients with large multifocal lesions may require gastric resection. Antrectomy may cause regression of ECL dysplasia and the small carcinoids, but antrectomy is not recommended because clinically significant lesions remain unaffected. Follow-up with repeated gastroscopy is suggested, and some evidence suggests that treatment with somatostatin analogues may prevent recurrence.

Type 2 gastric carcinoids associated with ZES in MEN1 patients: ECL cell hyperplasia occurs in 80% of patients with

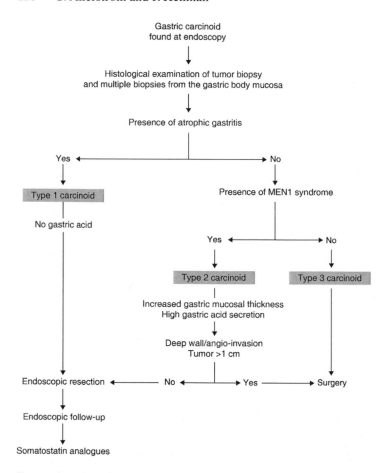

FIGURE 8.1. Gastric carcinoid found at endoscopy. Evidence of atrophic gastritis in the gastric body mucosa is a key point, allowing classification as a type 1 gastric carcinoid. If atrophic gastritis is not found, the patient should undergo screening for MEN1 syndrome (and ZES) (type 2 gastric carcinoid). If MEN1 is not diagnosed, the patient has the more aggressive type 3, sporadic gastric carcinoid (Reprinted from Delle et al., 2005. Copyright 2005. With permission from Elsevier).

the Zollinger-Ellison syndrome (ZES) secondary to Multiple Endocrine Neoplasia type 1 (MEN1); 15–30% of these patients develop carcinoids in the gastric body and fundus. In these patients, the mucosa thickness is increased in contrast to the atrophy of type 1 carcinoid neoplasms related to CAG, and the patients have increased gastric acid secretion (Fig. 8.1). A few patients (<1%) with sporadic ZES develop gastric carcinoids.

The type 2 gastric carcinoids are also often multicentric and small, but are generally larger (0.5–4 cm) than the type 1 gastric carcinoids, and occasionally are markedly larger. The malignant potential is intermediate between those of CAG-associated and sporadic gastric carcinoids. Lymph gland metastases occur in about 30% of patients and distant metastases in about 10%.

Surgical treatment should focus on removal of the source of the hypergastrinemia, most often by duodenotomy, local excision of duodenal gastrinomas, and lymphadenectomy of the periduodenal lymph nodes. The gastric carcinoids should be treated as type1 lesions with endoscopic mucosectomy for tumors <1 cm and liberal, focused excisions or gastric resection of larger neoplasms together with regional lymphadenectomy. Treatment with somatostatin analogues may decrease tumor growth, especially if hypergastrinemia has not been reversed by surgery, because gastrin drives the tumor growth.

Type 3 sporadic gastric carcinoids: Sporadic gastric carcinoid neoplasms account for 20% of gastric carcinoids. These neoplasms occur in non-atrophic gastric mucosa without endocrine cell proliferation. Determination of serum calcium and family history should be explored to exclude MEN1 (Fig. 8.1). The tumors, which are more frequent in males (mean age 50 years), are often large, with many exceeding 2 cm. Two-thirds of the lesions have infiltrated the muscularis, and 50% involve all layers of the gastric wall. Some sporadic gastric carcinoids occur in the antral or prepyloric region, although the majority are located in the body and fundus of the stomach. These neoplasms originate in the ECL cells, but when other cell types are present, the prognosis is less favorable. Regional lymph gland metastases occur in 20–50% of patients, and liver metastases will develop eventually in two-thirds of the patients. Sporadic carcinoids can have an atypical histology, with pleomorphism, mitoses, and often a higher Ki67 index. The atypical larger neoplasms >4 cm are frequently invasive and have an unfavorable survival.

An "atypical carcinoid syndrome" may be present in 5–10% of patients with sporadic gastric carcinoids. The syndrome is due to release of histamine and characterized by a patchy "geographic" flush, cutaneous edema, bronchospasm, salivary gland swelling, and lacrimation. Urinary measurement of the histamine metabolite MelmAA may serve as tumor marker, and patients may also have increases in urinary 5-HIAA values.

Sporadic gastric carcinoids require operative excision, often gastric resection combined with lymphadenectomy. Lesions larger than 2 cm, or those with atypical histology or gastric wall invasion, are managed most appropriately by gastrectomy. The 5-year survival is only 50%, but in patients with distant metastases, survival is only 10%.

Type 4 poorly differentiated gastric neuroendocrine tumors: Poorly differentiated (small cell) neuroendocrine carcinomas are highly malignant with extensive local invasion and usually with distant metastases at diagnosis. Atrophic gastritis is present in half of the patients. These neoplasms have a median size of approximately 4–5 cm, often appearing as ulcerating or fungating tumors. The prognosis is poor with a median survival of 8 months. These neoplasms are often not amenable to resection, although occasionally, surgical debulking together with chemotherapy may be considered in patients with mixtures of well- and poorly differentiated neoplasms.

Midgut Carcinoids

The small intestinal carcinoids are the most common (32%) among carcinoids and occur at a mean age of 65 years. Primary neoplasms are most prevalent in the terminal ileum, occurring typically as a small, submucosal tumor, sometimes visible only as a fibrotic, localized thickening of the intestine. Due to lymphatic spread, one-third of the patients have other multiple, smaller carcinoids in the small intestine. Mesenteric lymphatic metastases are frequent, even with the small neoplasms, and microscopic spread appears to be the rule rather than the exception. The metastases can often grow large and may be mistaken to represent the primary tumor. These neoplasms induce marked surrounding mesenteric fibrosis due to effects of local release of growth factors and serotonin. With progression, the mesentery often contracts, and with local fibrosis can cause intestinal obstruction, many times irreparable.

Symptoms: Carcinoids progress slowly and patients may have nonspecific abdominal pain or may even present (though less commonly) with features of carcinoid syndrome with diarrhea, discrete flush or intolerance for specific food or alcohol, even before the primary disease is overt. Bleeding can occur due to the submucosal location and small tumors. Abdominal pain attacks tend to increase in severity until bowel obstruction develops and patients require operative intervention. In nearly half of carcinoid patients, the diagnosis becomes evident only at operation for bowel obstruction. Extra-abdominal metastases may occur in the skeleton, the lungs, mediastinal and peripheral lymph nodes, ovaries, breast, and skin.

The classic carcinoid syndrome occurs eventually in 10–20% of patients presenting with flush, diarrhea, right-sided heart valve fibrosis, and bronchial constriction. The syndrome almost always occurs in the presence of extensive liver metastases or extensive retroperitoneal spread. Heart disease is a serious complication and may require valve replacement. Heart disease should be investigated by echocardiography before major abdominal surgery.

Diagnosis: Midgut carcinoids may be diagnosed by increased levels of the serotonin metabolite 5-HIAA in 24 h urine samples. While this finding is specific for carcinoids, it is present only in advanced disease and generally with evident liver metastases. Assay for plasma chromogranin A is less specific, but can provide earlier diagnosis, and is often used to monitor disease progression. Computed tomography (CT) often shows a pathognomonic finding of a mesenteric mass with radiating density (fibrosis)(Fig. 8.2). CT with contrast enhancement will demonstrate efficiently the presence of

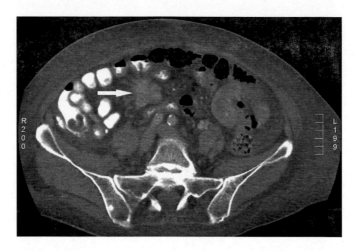

FIGURE 8.2. CT of mesenteric metastasis from midgut carcinoid.

mesenteric nodal metastases and retroperitoneal extension, as well as encasement of mesenteric vasculature. Octreoscan will detect carcinoid neoplasms with >90% sensitivity, and can determine metastatic spread, especially to extra-abdominal sites.

Histology: Needle biopsies from metastases, stained with chromogranin A and synaptophysin are used routinely to identify carcinoids; serotonin immune reactivity implies that the primary neoplasm is of midgut origin.

Early surgery: Midgut carcinoids can be suspected at laparotomy by the typical features of a small ileal tumor and large mesenteric metastases encircled by fibrosis. The primary neoplasm and metastases should be removed by wedge resection of the mesentery, and lymph node metastases should be cleared as efficiently as possible by dissection around the mesenteric artery and vein, aiming to preserve the vascular supply and limit the extent of intestinal resection. When a gross R-0 resection is achieved, patients may remain symptom-free for extended time periods, but carcinoids are tenacious, and recurrence within the liver and mesenteric nodes occurs in more than 80% of patients with long follow-up.

Advanced carcinoids: In patients with advanced carcinoid, treatment with long-acting somatostatin analogues and interferon-α can often provide efficient control of the carcinoid syndrome. During medical treatment, the mesenteric tumor and fibrosis will often progress and increase the risk of vascular and intestinal entrapment. Compromised mesenteric circulation and incipient venous ischemia contribute markedly to diarrhea, malnutrition, and malaise. Some patients have severe abdominal pain, weight loss, and malnutrition due to the extent of cachexia secondary to intestinal ischemia. Prophylactic resection and/or debulking of mesenteric metastases is recommended at an early stage, as the disease may be impossible to manage surgically at a later time. With careful technique(Fig. 8.3), mesenteric metastases should be dissected away from the mesenteric artery and vein, with preservation of the mesenteric circulation; avoiding a short bowel syndrome is crucial in these patients.

Prophylaxis against carcinoid crisis: Any operative intervention in patients with the carcinoid syndrome risks the induction of a carcinoid crisis with hyperthermia, shock, arrhythmia, excessive flush, or bronchial obstruction. Carcinoid crisis may be prevented by routine intravenous administration of the somatostatin analogue Octreotide (500 mg in 500 ml NaCl at 50 mg/h) before induction of anesthesia and during the operation.

Liver metastases: Liver metastases may be treated by resection or local ablation to reduce the tumor burden and release of bioactive peptides. Debulking procedures include conventional liver surgery and radiofrequency (RF) ablation; a few patients have been treated by liver transplantation, although this approach is not recommended. Other approaches include liver embolization and treatment with somatostatin analogues labeled with radioactive agents, in combination with other medical treatments.

The majority of patients with carcinoid syndrome have multiple and bilateral liver metastases and are best treated by medical management. Fewer than 10% have apparently solitary or dominant metastases amenable to resection. Hepatic

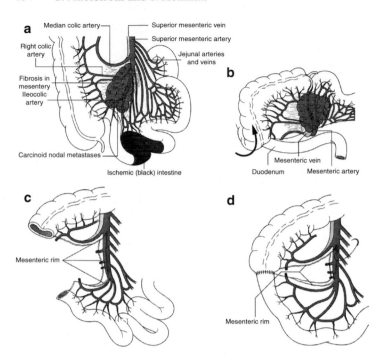

FIGURE 8.3. Resection of carcinoid primary tumor and mesenteric metastasis. (a) Mesenteric tumor may have extensive involvement of the mesenteric root. (b) Mobilization of cecum, terminal ileum, and mesenteric root allows the tumor to be lifted, approached posteriorly, and separated from duodenum and main mesenteric vessels, with preservation of intestinal vascular supply and intestinal length. (c, d) Bowel anastomosed and mesenteric defect repaired (Reprinted from Åkerström et al., 2006. Copyright 2006. With permission of Elsevier).

lobectomy or segmental liver resections are undertaken liberally for removal of such metastases and can be combined with wedge resections, enucleations, or RF ablation in the presence of other bilobar metastases with the idea of debulking. Two-stage liver resections combined with portal embolization in an attempt to trigger liver regeneration may reduce the risk of postoperative liver insufficiency.

Results of surgery and prognosis: Debulking surgery of mesenteric metastases in patients with incipient ischemia has been associated with long-term relief of abdominal symptoms and favorable 5-year survival of 90% in the absence of liver metastases. Significant symptom alleviation and long disease-free survival have been reported also after liver surgery in patients with the carcinoid syndrome if 90% of the tumor volume can be excised. Patients with inoperable liver metastases had 50% 5-year survival, and survival was 40% with inoperable liver and mesenteric metastases.

Appendiceal Carcinoids

Appendiceal carcinoids constitute 8% of carcinoids and are still the most common appendix neoplasm. These neoplasms are prevalent at autopsy, but are rarely of any clinical significance and may undergo spontaneous involution. The tumor can be expected in one per 300 appendectomies, but is usually only an incidental finding noted on histology of an excised appendix. The majority of appendiceal carcinoids are located at the tip of the appendix, and therefore, rarely cause appendicitis. Fewer than 10% are located at the appendix base. Patients are generally younger (mean age 40 years) than those with other carcinoids, and there is a female predominance. Children may also be affected. Metastases occur in only 4% of patients and more frequently in the younger patients.

The majority of appendiceal carcinoids have a favorable prognosis. Lesions without any vascular invasion that are confined to the appendiceal wall and are <2 cm in diameter (90% of appendiceal carcinoids) are cured by appendectomy. Lesions >2 cm or those with invasion of the mesoappendix, lymph node metastases, or residual tumor at resection margins, should be treated by right hemicolectomy and clearance of ileocecal mesenteric lymph nodes. Tumors at the appendiceal base require at least cecectomy to avoid residual tumor or recurrence, as they may originate in the colon rather than the appendix and thereby have more aggressive features. Lesions <2 cm confined to the appendiceal wall but with angioinvasion have uncertain malignant potential, and careful follow-up is required. An appendiceal carcinoid with liver or retroperitoneal metastases will only rarely cause the carcinoid syndrome.

Appendiceal carcinoids with mixed endocrine and exocrine (adenocarcinoma) features have been named goblet cell carcinoids. These aggressive neoplasms are more malignant, often with peritoneal metastases, and sometimes appearing as a mucinous adenocarcinoma of the ovary. This type of carcinoid does not express somatostatin receptors and cannot be visualized by OctreoScan. Treatment involves an aggressive right hemicolectomy and lymph node clearance, in combination with chemotherapy. For metastatic spread, aggressive operative reduction including oophorectomy and peritonectomy may be required, following recent guidelines for colorectal carcinomas.

Colon Carcinoids

Colon carcinoids are rare and account for only 10% of carcinoids. They present more often in older individuals (mean age 65 years). Carcinoids of the proximal colon are most common (50% occur in the cecum), and maybe associated, albeit infrequently, with the carcinoid syndrome, which does not occur with lesions in the distal colon or rectum. These carcinoids may be aggressive and have less well-differentiated histologic features. They tend to be large and exophytic, and have often reached conspicuous size (mean 4.9 cm) when detected, causing general systemic malignant symptoms, pain, and a palpable abdominal mass, but rarely bleeding. Metastases to lymph glands and the liver are present in the majority of patients at diagnosis. Treatment involves an aggressive hemicolectomy and lymph gland clearance. Due to their relatively slow growth, operative debulking may be indicated. Overall 5-year survival has been 40%, or slightly worse than for adenocarcinoma; survival is related primarily to tumor stage.

Poorly differentiated (small cell) neuroendocrine carcinoma occurs in the right colon and is frequently associated with an overlying adenoma or adjacent adenocarcinoma. Patients with these tumors generally have metastases at diagnosis and poor survival.

Rectal Carcinoids

Rectal carcinoids constitute 1–2% of all rectal tumors, and 11% of all carcinoids. They are somewhat more common in African-Americans than in Caucasians. The mean age is 55 years. Most rectal carcinoids occur 4–13 cm above the dentate line on the anterior or the lateral rectal wall. The majority are detected incidentally at endoscopy in asymptomatic patients, appearing as a solitary, typically yellowish, submucosal polyp <1 cm in diameter (Fig. 8.4). Locally advanced rectal carcinoids, >2 cm in diameter, appear in about 15%. The larger neoplasms may be associated with pain, change in bowel habits, constipation, and weight loss, and

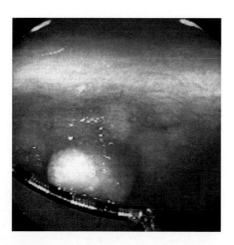

FIGURE 8.4. Rectal carcinoid polyp with typical yellowish color and submucosal location (Reprinted from McNevin and Read, 1998. With permission).

are occasionally also fixed to perirectal tissues, similar to adenocarcinomas. Multifocal tumors are rare. Tumors <1 cm rarely have metastases, tumors 1–2 cm in size have lymph node metastases in 4%, and distant metastases in 10–34%, with a higher risk of metastases when there is invasion of the muscularis layer. With tumors >2 cm, local and distant metastases occur in 67–100%, and virtually all patients eventually develop distant spread, most commonly in the liver. The carcinoid syndrome does not occur with rectal carcinoids.

Rectal carcinoids <1 cm can be removed safely by transanal excision and cauterization. Tumors measuring 1–2 cm should be investigated by transanal endosonography or magnetic resonance imaging. Absence of muscularis invasion or regional metastases justifies transanal endoscopic mucosectomy, whereas presence of either favors a more aggressive excision, generally by anterior resection and regional lymphadenectomy, which is also recommended in patients with tumors >2 cm without general dissemination. Due to lack of somatostatin receptors, OctreoScan is rarely of any value with rectal carcinoids, and chromogranin A is not often secreted, thus is not of use as a tumor marker. Resection of liver metastases may be considered in patients with limited spread of the more highly differentiated tumors, concomitant with chemotherapy. Proliferation is generally low in rectal carcinoids (Ki67 < 2%), although the larger or invasive tumors may have slightly higher Ki67 index and unfavorable survival. Overall 5-year survival for patients with distant metastases has been about 30%.

Selected Readings

Åkerström G, Hellman P, Hessman O (2006) Gastrointestinal carcinoids. In: Lennard TWJ (ed) Endocrine surgery. Elsevier, pp 163–198

Delle Fave G, Capurso G, Milione M, et al. (2005) Endocrine tumours of the stomach. Best Pract Res Clin Gastroenterol 19:659–674

Goede AC, Caplin ME, Winslet MC (2003) Carcinoid tumour of the appendix. Br J Surg 90:1317–1322

Modlin IM, Lye KD, Kidd M (2003) A 5-decade analysis of 13,715 carcinoid tumors. Cancer 97:934–959

McNevin MS, Read TE (1998) Diagnosis and treatment of carcinoid tumors of the rectum. Chir Int 5:10

Öberg K (1998) Carcinoid tumors: current concepts in diagnosis and treatment. Oncologist 3:339–345

Öhrvall U, Eriksson B, Juhlin C, et al. (2000) Method of dissection of mesenteric metastases in mid-gut carcinoid tumors. World J Surg 24:1402–1408

Vogelsang H, Siewert JR (2005) Endocrine tumours of the hindgut. Best PractRes Clin Gastroenterol 19:739–751

Wängberg B, Westberg G, Tylén U, et al. (1996) Survival of patients with disseminated midgut carcinoid tumors after aggressive tumor reduction. World J Surg 20: 892–899

Index